Ten Pitfalls in Intensive Care

Answer to the question on Book cover

Answer: This patient had a coarctation of the aorta. The upper arterial trace was from a radial line while the lower one was from a femoral catheter.

This patient needed surgery for a ruptured aneurysm that presented as a Subarachnoid Haemorrhage. The reason both lines were used was to ensure adequate perfusion pressures peri-operatively. The radial blood pressure (BP) was used to ensure a satisfactory cerebral perfusion pressure and the femoral BP to ensure adequate renal perfusion pressure.

Context: This is a young patient with Subarachnoid Haemorrhage. Subarachnoid haemorrhage is invariably due to a ruptured intracranial aneurysm & aneurysms at this age often have an associated congenital or genetic abnormality.

Differentials: There are two simultaneous arterial traces and the lower one has a much lower pulse pressure. Both have the same Diastolic BP (DBP) but the lower trace has a lower Mean BP (MBP) and Systolic BP (SBP).

Usually a decrease in pulse pressure suggests that the catheter tip is proximal or the trace is damped. But in either of these two situations, the MBP remains same & the SBP & DBP come closer to the MBP. Hence this is not a damped or simply a proximal trace.

The other differential is a stenotic lesion in the area between the two traces, as in the case of aortic coarctation. In such a situation, the DBP will be similar while the MBP & SBP will be lower in the femoral trace which is distal to the stenosis.

Ten Pitfalls in Intensive Care

Farhad N. Kapadia | Ritoo Kapoor

MACMILLAN
MEDICAL COMMUNICATIONS

ISBN: 978-93-80780-92-4

First Published in India 2016

Published by

Macmillan Medical Communications
An exclusive partner of nature publishing group.
3A, 5th Floor, DLF Corporate Park DLF Phase III,
Gurgaon–122002. India

Printed and Bound at Balaji Art, India.

MACMILLAN
MEDICAL COMMUNICATIONS

nature publishing group npg

ABOUT THE AUTHORS

FARHAD N. KAPADIA MD, FRCP, DA (UK), EDIC is a Consultant Physician and Intensivist at Hinduja Hospital, and a Visiting Consultant at Breach Candy, Cumballa Hill & Parsi General Hospitals in Mumbai, India.

He was the Founder President-Elect: Indian Society of Critical Care Medicine (ISCCM) and Chairman of the Societies' Education Program, Guidelines Committee & Research Committee. He is a Post Graduate Teacher in Intensive Care for the National Board of Examinations and the Indian College of Critical Care. He is also a Mumbai University Guide for M.Sc & PhD by Research in Applied Biology. He is actively involved in Research with approximately 100 international & 75 national publications & presentations. He has been the Primary, Co Investigator or Chief Coordinator in 13 international or national clinical studies. He regularly participates in national track and field athletics, marathons & ultra-marathons & plays saxophone in Jazz & Rock bands.

RITOO KAPOOR is a Consultant Intensivist and Anaesthetist based in Kent, UK. Apart from her NHS commitments in a District General Hospital she also has practicing privileges at BMI, Spire and Spencer Private Hospitals.

She gained her experience both as an intensivist and an anaesthetist in India, UK and Australia. She is actively involved in teaching and training at all levels and has designed and implemented an airway course for nurses on intensive care. She also leads on the nutrition care for hospitalised patients in her trust and is involved in the patient safety aspects of the same. She is a Medical performance assessor for the General Medical Council's fitness to practice procedures. She is a member of the editorial board of Intensive Care Monitor and is involved in critical care audit and research in her trust and has been an investigator in various trials.

Contact us at: tenpitfalls@gmail.com

TABLE OF CONTENTS

A Preview

The full table of contents is reproduced on page 221, but the reader is encouraged to identify the pitfall from the scenario before reading the title of the pitfall.

Introduction

Care of a critically ill patient in an Intensive Care Unit (ICU) requires some of the most technologically advanced aspects of modern medicine. It also raises complex ethical considerations, some of which have no right or wrong answers. The theme of this book is "Get the basics right and let the body then get on and heal itself."

A doctor is a man who writes prescriptions till the patient either dies or is cured by nature.

– John Taylor

In essence, the primary role of the intensivist is to keep the patient alive till the pathology is reversed and the body heals itself. The underlying physiology that results in healing is complex and incompletely understood.

The human body is centuries in advance of the physiologist, and can perform an integration of heart, lungs, and muscles which is too complex for the scientist to analyze.

– Roger Bannister Neuro-Physician and First athlete to do a sub 4 minute mile

Our ability to guess effective therapies has been very inadequate and not helped by the fact that the vast majority of trials have shown either lack of effect or shown harm. Staying "ahead of the game" and ensuring all avenues are covered, thus becomes paramount for the intensivist.

The care of a critically ill patient can be summarized in two working principles.

Working Principle 1: Reverse Primary Disease

Most critical illness is precipitated by sepsis, trauma, bleeding, or a major event like a myocardial infarction (MI), stroke or pulmonary embolism. The first working principle is to rapidly identify and limit or reverse the triggering disease.

Working Principle 2: Keep Patient Alive Using Standard ICU Life Support Techniques

Intensive care uses a lot of “default” therapies as a starting point where the prime goal is to keep the patient alive. These default therapies have evolved over the last few decades and are seen as standard treatment despite many being relatively untested. It is only recently that some of the standard therapies are being evaluated rigorously in randomized clinical trials.

Some of the standard treatments include protocols and algorithms for cardiopulmonary arrest; mechanical ventilation for a failing respiratory system; fluids, inotropes and vasopressors for a failing circulation; and renal replacement therapy for a failing kidney.

Once these are done, the patients will generally stabilize and show signs of recovery after which the life-support can be gradually withdrawn. During this period of life-support, high standards of nursing, infection control, appropriate nutrition and physiotherapy are required to prevent additional complications like infections and secondary sepsis, deep vein thrombosis (DVT), pulmonary embolism, gastrointestinal bleeds and skin breakdown due to pressure sores.

Intensivists have a vast armamentarium of therapeutic options in the care of their patients and many are relatively untested and used based on prior experience or on educated guesses. As mentioned earlier, most of the studies which have tested these therapies have been either negative or demonstrated harm. One therefore, needs to constantly update one’s knowledge and translate the newer findings into bedside practice. More often than not, this has meant giving up ineffective practices, rather than introducing newer effective ones. Evaluation of therapies has seen a shift of focus from physiological to clinically meaningful outcomes. Earlier, a medication would be viewed as effective if it attained a certain target, e.g. a systolic blood pressure of 90 mmHg. In recent trials the focus has been on, whether the drug in question decreased mortality or severity of illness as reflected by duration of illness and functional recovery. One should also remember that the physiology seen during a critical illness is the stressed response of the body. Many of the physiological parameters will therefore, fall outside the “normal” physiological range, and one should not automatically presume that normalization of physiological parameters are beneficial or desirable.

In order to deliver on the above two roles requires an adequate infrastructure. Part of this infrastructure is a set of pragmatic safety protocols, a clear system to ensure communication between all ICU and other medical personnel and relatives, a disciplined system of documentation, and also to ensure an adequate number of trained staff is present in the ICU.

Intensivists routinely deal with life threatening illnesses, anxious relatives and multiple colleagues from other specialties. The intensive care services consist of consultants, residents or trainees, nurses, physiotherapists and occasionally respiratory therapists. These ICU personnel have to communicate incessantly with each other and with other departments like the Emergency Department, the Operation Theatres, the Imaging Services, the Laboratory Staff and the Blood Bank. At every step of the way, there is a potential for delay or worse error. Many of these can be costly in terms of worsening clinical outcomes. In this maze of conflicting demands, it is important for the ICU to deliver a smooth and efficient service.

To paraphrase Google, the theme or motto of a Critical Care service could be "Don’t Be Sloppy".

Pitfall No. 1

Case Scenario

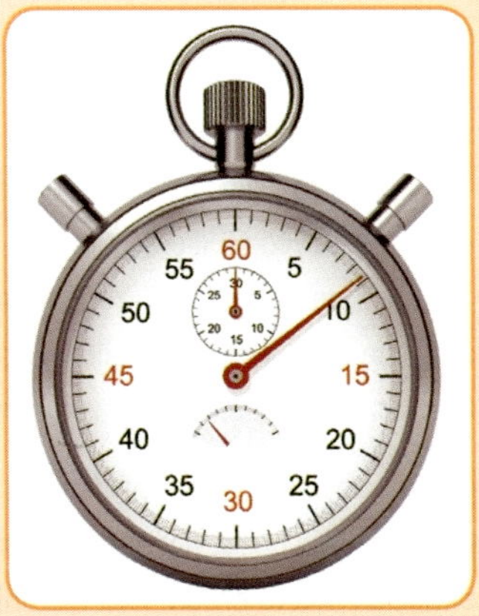

A 75-year-old gentleman presents to the emergency department with a 5 day history of fever and productive cough. He looks unwell, is tachycardic and tachypneic with a systolic blood pressure of 85 mmHg. Intravenous fluids are commenced and appropriate investigations sent. Right basal consolidation on the chest X-ray confirms a diagnosis of community-acquired pneumonia. After 2 liters of intravenous fluids the patient remains hypotensive. He is then transferred to the intensive care unit (ICU), and all standard monitoring and care are instituted. An internal jugular vein (IJV) central venous catheter (CVC) is inserted, and the central venous pressure (CVP) is 12 mmHg. As the hypotension persists, noradrenaline is commenced. The planned treatment drugs are written up and ordered. The patient continues to deteriorate and requires intubation and ventilation. The intubation requires 2 attempts and is a grade 3 intubation. Following little improvement over the next 2 days an ultrasound of the chest is performed and a pleural collection is confirmed. A pigtail catheter is therefore inserted and 300 mL of purulent material is drained.

What was the Pitfall?

Pitfall No. 1

Delay in Definitive Treatment

The pitfall was delay in definitive treatment of the primary disease. In this case, delay in administering the first dose of the antibiotic to a patient with septic shock. There was an additional delay in recognizing and draining an infected collection.

Time is Tissue.

In the above case scenario, it is not specified if and when the first dose of the antibiotic was given. It could have been in the emergency department, or immediately after transfer to ICU or even delayed till the scheduled time of a routine dose. In the case of antibiotics which are used only once or twice daily such as Ertapenem, a Carbapenem or Cefoperazone-Sulbactam, a third generation cephalosporin+β-lactamase inhibitor, the first dose can inadvertently be delayed by as much as 12-24 hours.

The single most important determinant of outcome in septic shock is probably the time in which the correct antibiotic is given, after the onset of hypotension. The initial treating physician has to ensure that the antibiotic is given before he/she leaves the patient. Also ensure that the *right drug*, the *right dose* and the *right route* are used. In this situation of septic shock, the initial dose should be a high-dose and it should be given intravenously. Avoid delays due to waiting for blood cultures to be collected, or waiting for drug-indent to be sent to pharmacy and the drug then reaching back from pharmacy. This implies that the emergency departments and ICUs must have a ready stock of culture bottles and routinely used antibiotics. If for any reason, there is a delay in getting blood cultures, it is preferable to give the first dose of antibiotics early, rather than delay awaiting culture collection.

It is important to give the full maximum dose of the antibiotic initially. Even if there is renal failure or hepatic dysfunction, the first dose should not be decreased, as the blood and tissue levels depend on the first dose being adequate. Later, doses can be appropriately reduced.

Plausibility: Septic Shock

The analogy of a match causing a forest fire is often used when describing the syndrome of infection leading to septic shock. Once the forest fire has spread, putting the match out will not reverse the situation. Most bacteria have a doubling time of 30 min. A simple calculation will demonstrate how important it is to give antibiotics early. If the doubling time is 30 min, by 5 hours the bacterial load will have increased > 1000 fold ($2^{10} = 1024$). By 48-50 hours, the bacterial load will have increased exponentially to $2^{100} = 1.3 \times 10^{30}$, (or 13 followed by 29 zeros). Bacterial and host factors will limit some of the growth, but the numbers do highlight exponential or scalable expansion of the septic process. These bacteria trigger a septic cascade, hemodynamic and micro-vascular changes, which result in hypoperfusion, cellular dysfunction and ultimately organ failure. The initial process takes place rapidly in the first few hours and it is at this point that antibiotics are most effective. The earlier the appropriate antibiotic is given, the lower would be the bacterial load and lesser triggering of the inflammatory and hemodynamic cascade. It is not surprising that delayed antibiotics will be much less effective than early antibiotics.

In certain situations, where the antibiotics cannot penetrate into the infected collection, antibiotics alone will not be enough. Once the patient has sufficiently stabilized, appropriate imaging must be done to identify infected collections or necrotic and devitalized tissue. These should be either drained percutaneously, if required under imaging, or if percutaneous drainage is not possible, surgical drainage should be done.

Evidence: Septic Shock

The main evidence for the efficacy of antibiotics comes from a paper by Kumar and colleagues.[1] The authors hypothesized that delay in administering the first dose of antibiotics after the development of hypotension would increase mortality in patients with septic shock. This retrospective cohort study was performed between July 1989 and June 2004, in fourteen intensive care units (four medical, four surgical, six mixed medical/surgical) and ten hospitals (four academic, six community) in Canada and the United States. They reviewed the medical

The single most important determinant of outcome in septic shock is the time in which the correct antibiotic is given, after the onset of hypotension.

records of 2,731 adult patients with septic shock and recorded the time between the onset of hypotension and the administration of the first dose of the appropriate antibiotic. Appropriate was defined as being the correct antibiotic based on the subsequent microbiological results. They found that if an antimicrobial effective for isolated or suspected pathogens was used within the first hour of documented hypotension, there was an associated survival rate of 79.9%. Each hour of delay in antimicrobial administration over the ensuing 6 hours was associated with an average decrease in survival of 7.6%. They also noted that only 50% of septic shock patients receive effective antimicrobial therapy within 6 hours of documented hypotension (Figure 1).

There have been other similar papers, but unfortunately, none are randomized trials. Given the magnitude of benefit seen in these observational trials, it seems unlikely that future investigators will get ethical clearance to randomize patients to delayed antibiotics.

The same author later reviewed the role of antibiotics in various clinical settings.[2] The focus was on varying efficacy in different infective situations. However, the literature is not uniform. Other authors too have shown that earlier antibiotics decrease mortality[3,4] but some have failed to find a mortality benefit.[5,6] It may be that this disparity is due to case mix. In observational studies where more patients were seriously ill primarily because of sepsis, early antibiotics decreased mortality. In some cohorts, the patients were mild to moderately ill, where the early administration was not so critical. Also, if the sepsis was part of an established Multi Organ Failure (MOF), then antibiotics alone may not have been enough to decrease mortality.

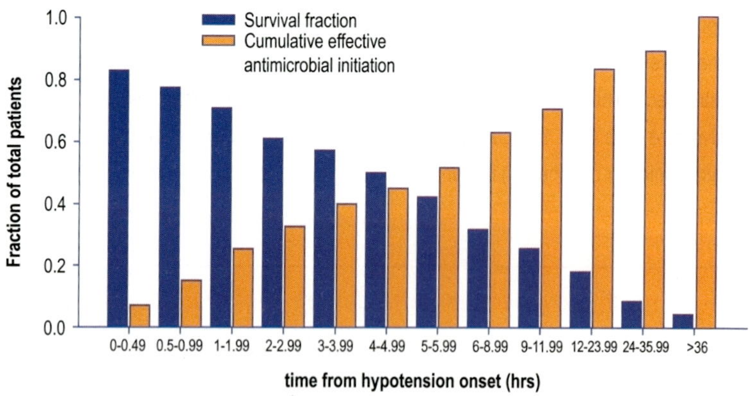

Figure 1. Effect of timing of antibiotic to mortality[1]
Source: *Crit Care Med* 2006;34:1589–1596.

It is currently inadvisable to give early high dose IV antibiotics in all potential or suspected infections, especially prior to development of systemic complications.

While early antibiotics are clearly beneficial in septic shock, the medical community needs to prevent widespread bacterial resistance secondary to antibiotic overuse. It should be clarified that early antibiotics are needed in patients presenting with sepsis and hypotension. It does not imply that all suspected infections without hypotension need immediate antibiotics. It also does not imply equal efficacy for recurrent sepsis in patients already in ICU with persisting MOF. In fact the BASIC study,[7] failed to show any pattern of antibiotic use associated with improved outcomes, among patients who develop bacteremia in ICU. Specifically, early versus late antibiotics and appropriate versus inappropriate antibiotics did not improve mortality. Similarly, a recent study failed to show an increase in mortality in surgical sepsis if inappropriate antibiotics were used.[8] One study in a surgical-trauma unit showed an increased mortality when early-aggressive antibiotic regimes were used.[9] Similarly, for new infections presenting to the emergency department without hypotension, it is unclear if early antibiotics will improve outcomes. It is currently inadvisable to give early high dose IV antibiotics in all potential or suspected infections, especially prior to development of systemic complications.

Early Definitive Treatment in Other ICU Emergencies

In some situations in the ICU, it makes little sense to "resuscitate" patients in the conventional sense of the term. All that is needed is definite immediate management. For example in patients on ICU with full monitoring, who develop Ventricular Fibrillation (VF) or Pulseless Ventricular Tachycardia (VT), it is better to immediately defibrillate them, rather than waste time on Airway Breathing and Circulation (ABC). Similarly, immediate defibrillation should be delivered as soon as a shockable rhythm is identified in any patient in cardiac arrest. In many instances, some ABC resuscitation would have been initiated before the VT/VF is identified on the monitor, and this should continue till the DC shock can be delivered. If cardioversion is not successful, then standard cardiopulmonary resuscitation (CPR) should be commenced or continued till the next DC shock is administered.

Similarly, if shock is due to a pericardial tamponade or a tension pneumothorax, there is little or no role in using invasive arterial and venous pressure monitoring and resuscitating with fluids and inotropes. Appropriate drainage of the pericardial fluid or pleural air is needed prior to any other resuscitative attempts. If the situation does not stabilize despite definitive therapy, it implies that some hypoperfusion injury has occurred. Conventional organ support may then be needed.

Early definitive therapy applies to any medical condition in which tissue viability is threatened. In acute coronary syndromes and ischemic strokes, early revascularization prevents or limits tissue damage. The same for surgical intervention in trauma or in raised intracranial pressure. In each of these conditions, delay in treatment results in worse clinical outcomes. Briefly discussed below is the current role for early treatment in other ICU emergencies.

Cardiopulmonary-Resuscitation

Among patients in cardiac arrest, if one assumes that CPR is done competently, the outcome depends on the duration of the arrest. This has two components, from point of cardiac arrest to starting CPR, a period of no flow, and from starting CPR to return of spontaneous circulation (ROSC), a period of low flow. The longer the time to ROSC, the worse the outcome. But, in that context, the cardiac arrest to CPR time is more important than the actual CPR to ROSC time.

Hypovolemia

Classic animal studies by Guyton showed that hypovolemic shock could be classified as reversible or irreversible. The body can compensate to a point, in terms of degree or duration of hypovolemia. Beyond that point, ischemic changes in tissues occur and replenishing the circulating volume will not change the outcome. Volume with fluid or blood replacement is therefore, the standard form of treatment of hypotension in most forms of shock. However, excess fluid resuscitation too may cause problems, and this will be discussed later with other pitfalls.

Acute Coronary Syndrome (ACS)

A large number of trials have shown that early revascularization has improved mortality in ACS. There are usually two options:

- Chemical revascularization with thrombolytic agents which have been shown to be effective in ST segment elevation myocardial infarction (STEMI).
- Mechanical revascularization with using primary angioplasty in myocardial infarction (PAMI) is beneficial in all forms of ACS, including those without ST-segment elevation

myocardial infarction (NSTEMI). Mechanical revascularization in the first few hours of an ACS has better recanalization rates, and is preferable to a chemical strategy, if the infrastructure can ensure revascularization early.

The situation becomes a little more complex when complications such as shock, respiratory failure or renal failure have occurred. Then, the timing of revascularization will depend on how quickly the patient can be stabilized with standard intensive care. Along with stabilization of the patient evaluation of the best therapy for the patient, be it a PCI (Percutaneous Coronary Intervention) or a CABG (Coronary Artery Bypass Graft), needs to be considered against the degree of physiological instability.

Trauma

The Advanced Trauma Life Support (ATLS) algorithms all stress the need for early therapy, whether it is fluid or blood replacement, or interventional or surgical procedures to stop bleeding.

Neurology

Raised intra cranial pressure (ICP) can result in herniation of one brain compartment into another and secondary ischemic changes. Rapid correction of this pressure whether with surgery or non-surgical measures prevents brain injury. Once the brain injury has occurred, relieving the raised ICP often leads to a surviving patient with a bad functional neurological state, potentially a fate worse than death. Similarly in an ischemic stroke, early recanalization with thrombolysis or neurointervention leads to better functional outcome and even mortality, compared to late therapy. In fact, late thrombolysis may lead to worse outcomes because of secondary hemorrhagic transformation in the infarcted area and further increase in ICP. Unlike ACS, the role of thrombolysis alone is less convincing. Most trials have shown a degree of functional benefit and often this is only seen after adjusting the data. The early mechanical intervention trials too were unsuccessful, but recent ones have demonstrated clear benefit. However, very few institutes have the infrastructure needed to deliver this form of therapy early enough to prevent brain injury.

Early definitive therapy applies to any medical condition in which tissue function or viability is threatened. Delay in treatment would result in worse clinical outcomes.

Etiology of a New Complication in an ICU Patient

The same approach is needed for a patient who is in ICU and develops a new complication, like hypotension, hypoxemia or distress. It is not enough to just increase the vasopressors or the FIO_2 or to sedate the patient. One must also run through a list of possible causes, like sepsis, pneumothorax, bleeding, reaction to drug or blood products, cardiac failure or pulmonary embolism. Failure to detect these will only allow a temporary stabilization with inotropes or increased FIO_2.

Conclusion: Pitfall 1-Delay in Definitive Therapy

It is vital to ensure that reversal of the etiology of the disease or new complication is done as rapidly as possible. As illustrated in the case scenario, it is not uncommon to find that the need to resuscitate and stabilize the patient results in delay of definitive therapy. As in this scenario, delay in administering antibiotics can be associated with worse clinical outcomes.

References

1. Kumar A, Roberts D, Wood KE, *et al.* Duration of hypotension before initiation of effective antimicrobial therapy is the critical determinant of survival in human septic shock. *Crit Care Med* 2006;34:1589–96.
2. Duane J Funk, Anand Kumar. Antimicrobial therapy for life-threatening infections: speed is life. *Crit Care Clin* 2011;27:53–76.
3. Yokota PK, Marra AR, Martino MD,*et al.* Impact of appropriate antimicrobial therapy for patients with severe sepsis and septic shock – a quality improvement study. *PLoS ONE* 2014;9(11):e104475.
4. Ferrer R, Martin-Loeches I, Phillips G,*et al.* Empiric antibiotic treatment reduces mortality in severe sepsis and septic shock from the first hour: results from a guideline-based performance improvement program. *Crit Care Med* 2014;42:1749–55.
5. Vilella AL, Seifert CF. Timing and appropriateness of initial antibiotic therapy in newly presenting septic patients. *American Journal of Emergency Medicine* 2014;32:7–13.
6. de Groot B, Ansems A, Gerling DH, *et al.* The association between time to antibiotics and relevant clinical outcomes in emergency department patients with various stages of sepsis: a prospective multi-center study. *Critical Care* 2015;19:194.
7. Corona A, Bertolini G, Lipman J,*et al.* Antibiotic use and impact on outcome from bacteremic critical illness: the BActeremia Study in Intensive Care (BASIC). *J Antimicrob Chemother* 2010;65:1276–85.
8. Davies SW, Efird JT, Guidry CA, *et al.* Does it matter if we get it right? Impact of appropriateness of empiric antimicrobial therapy among surgical patients. *Shock* 2014;42:185–91.
9. Hranjec T, Rosenberger LH, Swenson B, *et al.* Aggressive versus conservative initiation of antimicrobial treatment in critically ill surgical patients with suspected intensive-care-unit-acquired infection:a quasi-experimental,before and after observational cohort study. *Lancet Infect Dis* 2012:12:774–80.

Pitfall No 2

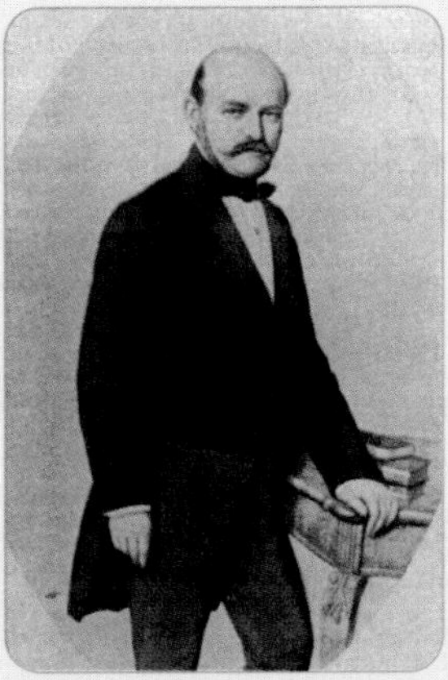

Who is this person?

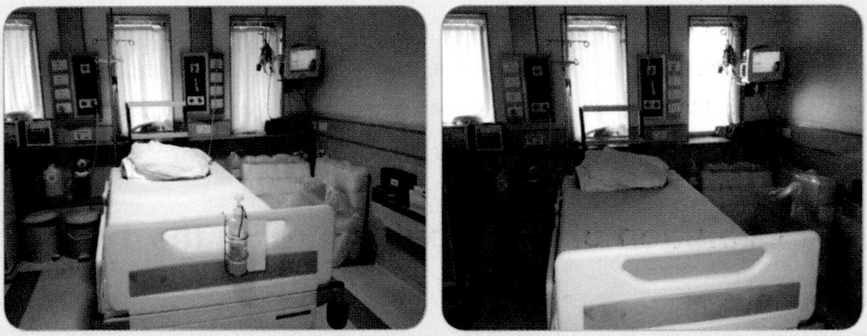

Spot the Difference

Pitfall No. 2

Inadequate Infection Control

Who is this person? Ignaz Semmelweis

Spot the Difference: No hand wash solution

Critically ill patients rarely die early in their illness from refractory shock or respiratory failure once they are adequately resuscitated with standard techniques. Some will rapidly improve and be weaned off life support. These are patients who are treated early, have rapidly & fully reversible primary illness, and minimal co-morbidity. Others may become refractory to treatment and die early. These are patients who are treated late, have poorly reversible or irreversible primary illness or have significant co morbidities. The majority however, will progress to varying degrees of multi-organ dysfunction. Then, after a period of stabilization many will make a slow recovery. These patients are at particular risk of secondary infections. Each episode of new sepsis or pneumonia increases the chance of death. After rapid eradication of the primary focus of illness, prevention of secondary sepsis is the most effective method of decreasing mortality and morbidity.

In the whole history of medicine, no single technique has improved clinical outcomes and mortality as much as simple hand washing and other infection control measures. The emergence of infection control could be seen in two phases. In the 19th Century, medical pioneers realized that infections could be transmitted via medical personnel, and it took some time for the message to get through to the medical community. Once the message was accepted, it took another century to become established practice. This led to further evolution of infection control from concepts to policies in the 20th and early 21st century.

The Evolution of Infection Control in the 19th Century

The 19th Century evolution is best told through the story of three pioneers, one U.S. Physician, one European Obstetrician-Gynecologist and one British Surgeon.

Oliver Wendell Holmes, Sr.

1809-94 *Poet, Physician and Essayist*

Oliver Wendell Holmes was born in Boston, educated at Harvard and later was a professor and dean at the same institute. Among his many writings, he published a paper, "The Contagiousness of Puerperal Fever" in *New England Quarterly Journal of Medicine and Surgery* in 1843. The essay hypothesized that the cause of the potentially fatal maternal puerperal fever, usually a few days after delivery, came from patient to patient contact via their physicians. This argument did not fit in with medical belief of the time as the germ theory of disease had not been postulated or discovered. He insisted that a physician, in whose practice even one case of puerperal fever had occurred, had a moral obligation to purify his instruments, burn the clothing he had worn while assisting in the fatal delivery, and cease obstetric practice for a period of at least 6 months.

Ignaz Philipp Semmelweis

1818-65

Semmelweis,[1] of Austrian-German extraction, was born in 1818 and later studied medicine in Pest and Vienna. He qualified in 1844 and later attained a Masters in Midwifery. He became a full assistant in 1846 at the Viennese School of Medicine, considered among the best in the world at that time. He noticed that the mortality in the medical school was always about three times that of the school of midwives even though the two divisions appeared identical. He noted that this increase was due to puerperal fever. Table 1 shows the difference in mortality in the two divisions. He wrote "There were heart-rending scenes when patients knelt down,

Table 1. Comparison of Mortality in Medical and Nursing division[1]

	First Division			Second Division		
Year	No. of cases	Deaths No.	%	No. of cases	Deaths No.	%
1841	3,068	237	7.7	2,442	86	3.5
1842	3,287	518	15.8	2,659	202	7.5
1843	3,060	274	8.9	2,739	164	5.9
1844	3,157	260	8.2	2,956	68	2.3
1845	3,492	241	6.8	3,241	66	2
1846	4,010	459	11.4	3,754	105	2.7
	20,042	1,989	9.92 say 9.9	17.791	691	3.38 say 3.3

wringing their hands, to beg for a transfer to the Second Division, having by a mistake on their part, applied for admission to the First Division........, the object being to avoid medical treatment, since they knew that medical treatment meant death." Many explanations were considered, but he stated "Everything remains without explanation, all is doubt and difficulty. Only the great number of the dead is an undoubted reality." He then describes his insight with the death of his friend Kolletschka, Professor of Forensic Pathology. "In the course of a post-mortem examination he was pricked in the finger by one of his pupils with a knife. Professor Kolletschka there upon became affected with lymphangitis and phlebitis in the same upper extremity, and he died from pleurisy, pericarditis, peritonitis and meningitis, and a few days before his death, metastasis occurred in one of the eyes. In the excited condition in which I was then, it rushed into my mind with irresistible clearness that the disease from which Kolletschka had died was identical with that from which I had seen so many hundreds of lying-in women die....."

He began, in May 1847, to use chlorinated lime with which every student was required to wash his hands before making an examination. The mortality fell from 12 to 3% in the first year of introduction of this practice. The next year it fell to 1.27% (45/3556), and for the first time, the medical division had a lower mortality than the nursing one. It is doubtful, in the whole history of medicine, if any single event had the impact of decreasing mortality as this simple technique did. Later in his career, he returned to his birthplace, Pest in Oct 1850. He introduced similar techniques. Soon after his appointment, the mortality rate in the old St Roque Hospital fell to less than 1%, while in other university clinics it was at times over 13%. This resulted in St Roque Hospital in Budapest being the first in the world to employ surgical antisepsis.

The mortality benefit in healthy young post-partum females was ~1 vs. 10-11%. This dramatic decrease was at minimal cost and no risk. Using the language of medical statistics, this translates to a Relative Risk Reduction of ~ 90%, an Absolute Risk Reduction of ~ 10%, a Numbers Needed to Treat of ~10 and an Odds Ratio of dying of ~ 0.09.

This outstanding success story should be part of the curriculum of all medical courses, not only to highlight medicines' greatest success story, but to highlight that the community needs

---

In the whole history of medicine, no single technique has improved clinical outcomes and mortality as much as simple hand washing and other infection control measures.

---

to be open to new pioneering ideas. Semmelweis was not so lucky. His first paper had one immediate effect, making his chief, Professor Klein, his critic and enemy. His concepts were widely debated and mostly rejected. This rejection dogged him in his later appointment. His concepts did gain some acceptance in England and Ireland though. Edward Murphy wrote a favorable paper in the Dublin Quarterly Journal of Medical Science in August 1857. The German professors publicly stated that the doctrine was discredited and universally rejected, and he responded with the publication of a book in 1861, "The Cause, Nature and Prevention of Puerperal Fever." This is now universally regarded as a major medical classic. However, he faced further isolation and development of mental disease, and at age 47, he was admitted to a mental asylum in Vienna, where, he pricked his hand doing a post-mortem, and 13 day later, he died of sepsis.

...in the whole history of medicine there is only one Semmelweis in the magnitude of his services to Mankind, and in the depth of his sufferings from contemporary jealous stupidity and ingratitude.

– Sir William Sinclair (1909)

Joseph Lister

1827-1922

Despite the work of Oliver Wendell Holmes and Ignaz Semmelweis, hospitals continued to practice surgery under unsanitary conditions. Around this time, the concept of germs as a cause of disease was first considered. The French chemist Louis Pasteur showed that rotting and fermentation could occur under anaerobic conditions, if micro-organisms were present. Pasteur suggested three methods to eliminate the micro-organisms responsible for gangrene: filtration, and exposure to heat, or to chemical solutions.

Joseph Lister was educated in London and later became professor of surgery in Glasgow. He became aware of Pasteur's work and explored the use of chemical solutions to treat human tissue. In August 1865, Lister discovered the antiseptic properties of carbolic acid by applying the solution onto the wound of an 11-year-old boy who had sustained a compound fracture. After four days, he noted that no infection had developed, and after a total of 6 weeks noted that the boy's bones had fused back together, without the danger of suppuration. He then published a series of articles on the Antiseptic Principle and Practice of Surgery in *The British Medical Journal.*

Like Semmelweis, he noticed that midwife-delivered babies had a lower mortality rate than surgeon-delivered babies, correctly attributing this difference to the fact that midwives tended to wash their hands more often than surgeons, and that surgeons would often go

In the late 19th century, with the development of germ theory by Louis Pasteur and its subsequent application to surgical sterility by Joseph Lister, surgeons were able to operate with a substantially reduced risk of infection.

directly from one surgery, such as draining an abscess, to delivering a baby. He instructed surgeons under his responsibility to wear clean gloves and wash their hands before and after operations with 5% carbolic acid solutions. Instruments were also washed in the same solution and assistants sprayed the solution in the Operation Theatre.

The germ theory of disease slowly gained acceptance, and it became universally acknowledged that infection could be better avoided by preventing bacteria from getting into wounds in the first place. This led to the rise of sterile surgery, with Lister being called "The Father of Modern Anti Sepsis."

The Evolution of Infection Control in the 20th and 21st Century

The 20th and 21st Century saw a major shift in infection control. Around the turn of the century, hospitals or the so called institutions were a crowded mess of sick individuals and hospital acquired infections. Healthcare Associated Infections (HCAI), as we know them today, were rampant. Instead of being a place to get well they almost became a source of illness themselves. Following, the introduction of antibiotics and an understanding of asepsis, these institutions then evolved into hospitals which helped patients get better. The infection control focus changed from techniques to implementation.

Prevention of HCAI and infection control measures have now been around for nearly 70 years in some shape or form. In the UK, this took the shape of supervising officer for infection control in 1941, the establishment of a committee to oversee infection control measures in 1944 as recommended by the British Medical Research Council (MRC) and an infection control nurse in 1959.[2] While the 1930s–1950s were dominated by streptococcal infections, the late 1950s and the 1960s saw a shift towards staphylococcal infections and by 1985 this had led to the appointment in 89% of NHS hospitals of an infection control nurse and in 100% a doctor, usually a consultant microbiologist who became the infection control doctor.[3]

In the 1980s, the Centre of Disease Control in the USA initiated the Study on the Efficacy of Nosocomial Infection Control (SENIC) to evaluate the approaches to infection control and surveillance. Following publication of their report, studies from other parts of the world started appearing. In the UK, a national prevalence survey was commenced in 1980 and has since delivered 4 reports, the last one being in 2011. About the same time as surveillance was being looked at, there was also an emerging trend that looked at the financial implications of Health Care Acquired Infection (HCAI). A study published in 1999 estimated the cost of HCAI in the National Health Service (NHS) to be almost £1 billion a year, with patients remaining in hospital an extra 3.6 million days.[4] This eventually led to the clinical governance framework and the statutory responsibility for infection control to be introduced by the Department of Health.

In 2000, the publication of the report by the National Audit Office (NAO)[5] into the incidence of HCAI caused a media frenzy which also fuelled public interest in the topic. This led to a focus on clean hospitals as the public perceived clean hospitals as being safe hospitals. The government obliged by introducing guidelines, and inspections to ensure compliance with the guidelines. This gave impetus to research into infection control. But, the research focus was contamination which didn't automatically translate to cross infection. What followed was the development of the evidence based guidelines for preventing HCAI in the NHS (EPIC). This led to an increase in surveillance but the follow up report from the NAO in 2004 continued to be critical and still concluded that there was patchy implementation of the infection control guidelines.[6] The Department of Health then introduced its action plan, *Towards Cleaner Hospitals and Lower Rates of Infection* which re-emphasized the importance of hand hygiene and environmental cleanliness. This was the first step towards the introduction of targets to reduce HCAI. Although by 2008, there was a 57% reduction in MRSA bloodstream infections and a 41% reduction in Clostridium difficile infections[7] HCAI in terms of overall incidence didn't show a statistical difference between that in 2006 versus that in 2011.[8] All this was happening in the media glare which in some ways influenced policy change towards a popular common sense approach rather than scientific evidence.

Hand hygiene thus became one of the most heavily regulated policies for infection control. But even today, it does not have 100% compliance. A study looking at hand hygiene frequency in ICU estimated that in order to comply with all contacts, a health care worker would need to decontaminate their hands in excess of 120 times in a given shift,[9] a clearly impossible

In the 20th century, infection control focus changed from techniques to implementation, with the use of chemotherapy and prophylactic antibiotics.

task. In some ways decontaminating hands has become the main focus of infection control measures rather than one part of it.

Then came the "Bare below the elbows" (BBE) dress code, introduced by the Department of Health, UK, in 2007 which banned long sleeves, jewellery and wristwatches. The aim was to improve the quality of hand hygiene and prevent bacterial transfer from cuffs of long sleeve white coats that were traditional attire for doctors. Studies looking at contamination of doctors' coats found cuffs and pockets to be the most contaminated with nearly a quarter harboring staphylococcus aureus. Surgical specialties had a higher incidence as compared to medical specialties.[10] But a study conducted in 2010 concluded that BBE did not improve the quality of hand hygiene and neither did it prevent HCAI.[10]

In 2011, the prevalence of HCAI in NHS hospitals was 6.4%, down from 8.2% in 2006 yet the highest prevalence was in patients in ICU (adult 23.4%, pediatric 14.7% and neonatal 13.1%) although, they only accounted for 9.4% of the total HCAI detected.[8] Even though the advancement in medical technologies and better research into preventative medicine has seen a dramatic reduction in HCAI, it continues to remain the bane of many hospital admissions. This could be attributed to the increase in invasive monitoring, invasive procedures, immunosuppressive treatments, use of broad-spectrum antibiotics etc. Add to this mix an ageing population, a drive towards efficiency and the financial implications and suddenly HCAI impact most hospital delivered care.

Infection Control in Contemporary ICU

A primary responsibility of the ICU team is to ensure minimal secondary infections in their vulnerable patients. At this point, it is worth stressing that infections in ICU are partly due to cross contamination, and partly due to decreased host protective immune responses. In certain epidemic situations such as the SARS epidemic or the H1N1 epidemic, infection control to prevent cross infection is critical, to the point of near total isolation of the patients and maximal infection control precautions for all ICU personnel caring for that patient. Keeping these isolation rooms at a slightly negative pressure from the rest of the ICU prevent these highly transmissible infection from spreading to the main ICU. In other situations like a multi-drug resistance tuberculosis (TB) patient too, these near total infection control policies are needed. Similarly, severely immune suppressed patients with e.g. bone marrow transplants have to be completely isolated and once again ICU personnel need to follow maximum infection control procedures. Keeping these isolation rooms at a slightly positive pressure from the rest of the ICU prevents the ICU flora from reaching these vulnerable patients. However, these maximal infection control policies are unnecessary in the average

ICU patient with common ICU diseases such as sepsis, trauma or surgical multi-organ failure. Here, a clean environment and standard infection control protocols need to be followed. Unlike an operation theatre that needs to be kept sterile with high quality air filters and multiple air exchanges, the ICU environment simply needs to be clean and hygienic. It is often said that patients should be kept out of ICU or moved out of ICU because "ICU is a place where one gets infections." This is silly. Infections occur because patients are vulnerable. Stable patients who are kept in ICU or a high dependency unit (HDU) purely for observation almost never get infected. Similarly, personnel working in ICU for years or decades too never get infected by the standard ICU organism, because their general health is enough to prevent these infections. The same applies to patients' relatives and visitors.

It is useful for ICUs and health care service providers to have clear, simple, lucid and pragmatic protocols and policies for infection control. An example of such a protocol and policy is shown in Figure 1.

Infections from the surrounding are called exogenous while those from the colonizers within the patient are called endogenous infections.

Endogenous Infection Prevention

Probably, the most important strategy to limit endogenous infections is to shorten the duration of the critical illness. This is best achieved by rapid correction of the primary disease and rapid resuscitation. Established protocols including daily awakening with sedation breaks promote early weaning and extubation. Other techniques to prevent endogenous infections have had variable success. These include semi-recumbent body position in ventilated patients, early enteral nutrition and immune enhancing feeds, tight sugar control, use of oral rather than nasal endotracheal and gastric tubes, and glottic aspiration in intubated patients. Oral chlorhexidine has been recommended to decontaminate the upper airway and selective decontamination of the digestive tract to lower, and limit the potential pathogens in the bowel from causing endogenous infections. All these techniques have been studied to various

---

The most important strategy to limit endogenous infections is to shorten the duration of the critical illness, by rapid resuscitation and prompt correction of the primary disease.

---

degrees with the evidence showing benefit in some papers and harm in others. A couple of examples: In the early tight sugar control studies,[12] infections were reduced but the largest study to date[13] showed an increased mortality associated with tight sugar control. Similarly, though the use of chlorhexidine is recommended in many guidelines, a meta-analysis[14] on the use of chlorhexidine to decontaminate the oropharynx showed no benefit in non-cardiac patients and minimal benefit in cardiac surgical patients.

Exogenous Infection Prevention

Exogenous infections could enter the patients through various routes and personnel. It helps to have pragmatic infection control protocols which focus on care of the ICU, care of the bed space, care at point of staff contact with patient, care of indwelling devices and care of external devices. Many of these policies and recommendations are based on experience and reasonable theoretical considerations, and most are not backed up by evidence to show superiority to alternative approaches. Two of the more important of these recommended practices are to wash hands prior to contact with any invasive devices, and to avoid touch contamination by using maximum barrier precautions when doing invasive procedures.

Unfortunately, some of these unproven practices can gain cult status and then become impossible to disprove or dislodge. The NHS, in UK, has multiple unproven policies regarding the use of wrist watches, ties, "bare below the elbows", no white coats etc. and despite being humorously questioned[15] are unlikely to disappear any time soon. This highlights a problem when policy makers are not familiar with the subject or the methodology of science. These policy makers are often incapable of distinguishing a hypothesis from a conclusion. As a result, they give equal weight to a plausible idea and a proven practice. Once these policies are laid down, it becomes impossible for practicing physicians to not follow them, even if they feel the policy is useless or harmful.

Washing hands prior to contact with patient or with invasive devices, and maximum barrier precautions to avoid touch contamination during procedures are strongly recommended for prevention of exogenous infections.

Common infections that are prevented with infection control measures are ventilator associated pneumonia, vascular catheter associated blood stream infections, and catheter associated urinary tract infection

Impact of Infection Control on Clinical Outcomes

The examples of reduction in mortality secondary to infection control in Semelweiss' and Lister's time are dramatic, but the situation is not so straightforward in today's ICUs. When patients already have MOF and other multiple comorbidities, part of the problem is the reduced host immune response, and certain bacteria, which are normally only potentially pathogenic, can invade the host and cause infections. In these situations, patients probably die with, rather than of, secondary infections. The common infections that are prevented with infection control measures are ventilator associated pneumonia (VAP), vascular catheter associated blood stream infections (CRBSI), and catheter associated urinary tract infection (CAUTI). Unfortunately, the diagnosis of each is not black and white and different diagnostic criteria result in different infection rates. Also, the rates are sometimes calculated per day and sometimes per patient, making it difficult to benchmark. Despite this, benchmarking against a fixed standard is a useful way of knowing the efficacy of the infection control protocols and practices in a given ICU. Most studies evaluate the efficacy of infection control practices to infection, and not to clinical outcomes. There are no large head to head studies that show a clear mortality benefit by preventing infections in ICU patients with MOF. Rather, there is a calculated "attributable mortality", which may be up to 35% in the case of VAP. Despite this lack of unequivocal evidence of a mortality benefit with infection control especially in those who are already critically ill, it is worth being obsessive about implementing standard and pragmatic infection control practices for all patients in ICU.

Conclusion

Infection control is one of the greatest, if not the single greatest achievement of medicine in the last 2-3 centuries. ICU patients are vulnerable and can get infected by cross contamination with ICU organisms and also with their own endogenous bacteria. Strict infection control practices focused on sterility at the point of contact with the patient and with indwelling

Figure 1. An example of an Infection Control Protocol and Policy for an ICU

- **Components of Protocols**
  - Care of the ICU
  - Care of the Bed space
  - Care at point of staff contact with patient
  - Care of indwelling devices
  - Care of external devices
- **Role of ICU Director**
  - Active in Infection Control Committee
  - Regular surveillance of infection trends
  - Limit traffic in ICU
  - Antibiotic policies and prevention of antibiotic abuse
  - Training and awareness on part of all ICU personnel
  - Compliance with protocols by visiting consultants
  - Uniformity of epidemiological data
- **Hand wash Solution Options**
  - Self-drying solution
    - 70% Alcohol +/- 0.5% Chlorhexidine
  - Soap and Water
- **Sterilizing Solution Options**
  - Detergent and water
  - 11% H_2O_2 + 0.01% Silver Nitrite
  - Formaldehyde + Glutaraldehyde
  - 2% Glutaraldehyde
  - 5% Hypochlorite diluted (75 mL in 12 L of water) to ensure > 100 ppm of Chloride
- **Care of the ICU**
  - General Cleaning of ICU: Clean thrice daily + as needed
  - Thorough machine clean once weekly

- Clean with disinfectant
  - Dirty Utility Room
    - Cold +/- hot water and disinfectant availability
    - Adequate dry stand and shelf space
    - Cups, bedpans, urinals etc. to be kept dry

- **Care of the ICU: What's no longer recommended**
  - Fumigation
  - Changing of footwear
  - Restricting relatives visiting times
  - Protective clothing
- **Care of the Bed space**
  - Hand wash solutions / basin at each bedside
    - Self drying solution (Alcohol (70% +/- Chlorhexidine)
  - Separate AMBU bag, face mask and stethoscope per bedside
    - Clean with spirit for each new patient
  - Bed space cleaned before arrival of new admission + As required
  - Clean floor x 3 daily + As required
  - Walls cleaned two weekly + As required
  - Glass partitions cleaned daily
  - Curtains (partition) changed weekly + As required
  - Curtains (windows) changed two weekly + As required
  - Linen changed daily + As required
- **Care of Patient Contact**
  - Wash hands before patient contact
  - Re-wash prior to contact with
    - Vascular catheter and its connections
    - Tracheal tube and its connections
    - ICP monitor
  - Change patients position regularly

        - Prevents hypostatic pneumonia, bedsores
    - Air bed if longer than 2-3 day of immobility
- **Doing a Procedure**
    - Separate trolley
    - Do not move a common trolley from bedspace to bedspace
    - Separate trolley cleaned and loaded before a bedside procedure is done
    - Surface cleaned with disinfectant (Microshield or Sterillium)
    - Surface completely covered with a sterile drape
- **Care of Indwelling Devices** (Vascular catheters, Urinary catheters,Tracheal tubes, ICP catheter)
    - Appropriate sterile precautions for insertion
    - Wash hands before (and after) contact
    - Minimal disconnection
    - Protective plastic sheath if appropriate
    - Appropriate dressing and care protocol
    - Avoid "routine" changes
- **Care of External Devices** (IV sets, Infusions and Transducers)
    - Total Parentral Nutrition (TPN) through separate dedicated set/port
    - Fluids and drug infusions changed after 24 hours
    - Infusion set changed every 24 hours for TPN and every 3 days for other fluids
    - Consider use of disposable equipment
    - Ventilator Circuit and tubing
        - Disposable circuits if feasible
        - No routine change of circuit, catheter mount or stericath
        - HMEF at Y-connection for all patients
        - HMEF to be changed 24-48 hours
        - HMEF not to be removed from circuit except at time of changing

devices will limit exogenous infections. Rapid reversal of primary illness and resuscitation will allow quick recovery and limit the potential for endogenous infections. Clear protocols and policies help in implementing these infection control practices.

References

1. Elek SD. Semmelweis commemoration. Semmelweis and the oath of Hippocrates. *Proc R Soc Med* 1966;59:346–52.
2. Forder AA. A brief history of infection control – past and present. *SAMJ* 2007;97 No:1161–64.
3. Howard AJ. Infection control organization in hospitals in England and Wales, 1986. Report of a survey undertaken by a Hospital Infection Society working party. *J Hosp Infect* 1988;11:183–91.
4. Plowman R, Graves N, Griffin M, *et al.* The socio-economic burden of hospital acquired infection. London: Public Health Laboratory Service. 1999.
5. National Audit Office. The management and control of hospital acquired infections in acute NHS trusts in England. London: The Stationery Office. 2000.
6. National Audit Office. Improving patient care by reducing the risk of hospital acquired infection: a progress report. London: The Stationery Office. 2004.
7. National Audit Office. Reducing Healthcare Associated Infections in Hospitals in England. London: The Stationery Office. 2009.
8. Hopkins S, Shaw K, Simpson L. English National Point Prevalence Survey on Healthcare-associated Infections and Antimicrobial Use: Preliminary Data. 2011. Health Protection Agency.
9. McArdle F, Lee R, Gibb A, *et al.* How much time is needed for hand hygiene in intensive care? A prospective trained observer study of rates of contact between healthcare workers and intensive care patients. *J Hosp Infect* 2006 ;62: 304–10.
10. Wong D, Nyek K, Hollis P. Microbial flora on doctor's white coats. *BMJ* 1991;303:1602–04.
11. Farrington R, Rabindran J, Crocker G *et al.* "Bare below the elbow" and quality of hand washing: A randomized comparison study. *J Hosp Infect* 2010;74: 86–88.
12. Van den Berghe G, Wouters P, Weekers F, *et al.* Intensive insulin therapy in critically ill patients. *N Engl J Med* 2001;345:1359–67.
13. The NICE-SUGAR Study Investigators. Intensive versus Conventional Glucose Control in Critically Ill Patients. *N Engl J Med* 2009;360:1283–97.
14. Klompas M, Speck K, Howell MD, *et al.* Reappraisal of routine oral care with chlorhexidine gluconate for patients receiving mechanical ventilation: systematic review and meta-analysis. *JAMA Intern Med* 2014;174:751–61.
15. Rhys Clement. Is it time for an evidence based uniform for doctors? *BMJ* 2012;345:e8286.

Pitfalls No. 3, 4 & 5

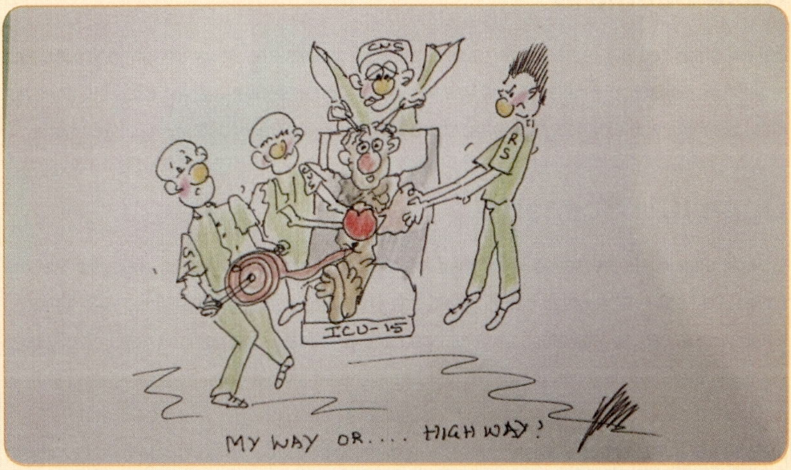

Cartoon by Dr. C Balakrishan MD. Consultant Rheumatologist, Hinduja Hospital, Mumbai

Pitfalls No. 3, 4 & 5

Case Scenario

Patient stabilizes but is not better over the next 2 weeks and he is still on inotropes and requiring mechanical ventilation. He has repeated spontaneous breathing trials but does not meet weaning and extubation criteria, and a percutaneous tracheostomy has been done.

Open ICU Scenario

Multiple specialists are called in for their input. The respiratory physician suggests that the patient be kept in a negative balance and dry. The urine output is maintained with diuretics but the previously normal blood urea nitrogen and creatinine start rising. A nephrologist then suggests that the fluids be increased, that the ICU start "Renal dose dopamine" and plan to dialyze the patient. The hemoglobin (Hb) is low at 9 gm/dL (90 g/L) and the PT and PTT are prolonged. The D-dimer is raised and the hematologist suggests blood and blood products to keep Hb > 10 gm/dL (100 g/L) and to correct the abnormal coagulation parameters. The albumin is 2 gm/dL (20 g/L) and the gastroenterologist recommends that the ICU replace albumin and start total parenteral nutrition (TPN). The patient develops atrial fibrillation (AF) and the cardiologist starts amiodarone and anticoagulation. He has recurrent episodes of fever and the imaging and cultures do not show a new infection, but an infectious disease consultant feels that it would be worthwhile escalating the antibiotics and also include MRSA and antifungal cover with preferably one of the newer echinocandins.

A few facial twitches are noted, a neurologist is called and phenytoin is added. An EEG and MRI are requested. The EEG only shows slowing without seizure activity, but the neurologist feels it would be safer to add a second drug, so Lacosamide is added.

Closed ICU Scenario

Four intensivists rotate with two of them covering the first week and the other two covering the second week. During the first intensivist's cover, this and all patients get pressure control ventilation (PCV), liberal packed red blood cells (PRBC) and very early nutrition. During the second intensivist's period, this patient and most other patients get albumin and multiple antibiotics. During the third intensivist's stint, this and all patients get a spontaneous breathing trial on pressure support ventilation (PSV) on a ventilator, (while others use a T-piece trial). During this stint restless patients are tied to the bed and liberally sedated, while the other three do not use physical restraints and they use minimal judicious sedation. The fourth intensivist does not change any orders and leaves all new decisions to other specialists and colleagues.

Question: What are the Pitfalls?

The Pitfalls are poor knowledge and implementation of Evidence Based Medicine.

The above two scenarios highlight a near universal problem in ICUs: varying practice patterns by different physicians. The best way to improve uniform yet effective care is for all treating physicians to agree to practice evidence based medicine (EBM), to focus on clinical outcomes and to avoid using too many unproven therapies. It is now necessary for practicing physicians to be updated with the peer reviewed medical literature, and also develop the skills to interpret the literature, especially the methodology of the major studies which are usually RCTs and meta-analysis using mortality as the primary outcome. Practitioners also need to be willing to give up disproved practices. Certain "routine" aspects of ICU care such as the use of the Swan-Ganz catheter, renal dose dopamine and liberal blood transfusions have become less common, as emerging literature has shown lack of any clinical benefit.

The practice of medicine has been described as both a science and an art. Unfortunately, this "art" aspect is sometimes seen as a license to ignore all scientific principles and practice in any way one presumes to be correct. An unwillingness to constantly re-evaluate ones practices and modify them can lead to stagnation, and can deny the patients benefit of new knowledge. It is imperative to at least know all the new data from the recent and current large RCTs which show impact on clinical outcomes. If one chooses not to believe them, one should at least have clear scientific reasons for doing so. There is a saying in Jazz music: to break the rules, you first have to know the rules. Similarly, in the practice of medicine, to reject conclusions from data, one should first fully know and understand the data. Rejecting conclusions from data alone because it does not fit one's preconceptions and practices will lead to poor patient care in the long run. It is helpful to have a teaching program and regularly participate in conferences and updates, as these make one review and consider changing entrenched practices that may no longer be valid.

In the appendix, there is a discussion on the underlying principle of evidence-based medicine and a simple plan for how one should read a randomized clinical trial (RCT) or a meta-analysis.

When using data from trials to treat intensive care patients, one should avoid a few potential errors. One important consideration is, if the study was done on intensive care patients in

Physicians need to be updated with peer reviewed medical literature, and develop skills to interpret RCTs and meta-analysis of major trials using mortality as primary outcome.

When using data from trials to treat intensive care patients, one important consideration is to clarify that the study was done on intensive care patients and not on stable medical surgical patients.

the first place. For example many studies done for patients with Atrial fibrillation (AF) or cardiac failure have been done on ambulatory patients, and it is unclear if the ICU patient will show a similar benefit. It is well accepted that patients with chronic AF will decrease the stroke risk with the use of anticoagulants. But there is no clarity on whether the patient who develops a new onset AF in ICU will have a similar benefit. Even if there is a benefit, there is no clarity as to how early or late one should start anticoagulation. Beta-blocking agents and drugs such as ivabradine have been shown to offer some benefit to ambulatory patients with cardiac failure, but using them in the decompensated cardiac failure patient in ICU may make the situation worse.

The next issue is how to deal with trials which have opposite results. Here one of two patterns generally emerge. One, initial trials are small and positive and later large trials are negative. Two, after a series of negative trials, one RCT shows unequivocal benefit.

Initial trials positive and subsequent ones negative: In such a situation, the large trial is more likely to reflect the actual efficacy of the drug. The use of tight sugar control and albumin are examples of this.

Another reason is that the care of patients in the control arm may improve over the years as the general standard of care improves. The Early Goal Directed Therapy trials (EGDT) highlight this. The first trial by Rivers *et al.*[1] was clearly beneficial and the second[2] questionably beneficial. The three large subsequent trials ProMISe, ARISE and ProCESS[3–5] were all negative, but tellingly had a much lower mortality in both treatment and control patients. The simplistic explanation is that the practice of early antibiotics and resuscitation became standard, at least in the participating centres, and hence, the outcomes were better.

Initial trials negative and subsequent ones positive: Two recent examples highlight this: the role of thrombolysis and neurointervention in thrombotic stroke and the use of prone position ventilation in severe ARDS.

The use of thrombolytic agents and neuro-intervention in ischemic stroke is a good example. The initial thrombolysis trials (6 RCTS) from the 1990s,[6–11] showed some functional benefit, but the results were unconvincing to many practicing clinicians. A later trial (IST-3) in 2012[12] covered more than 3000 patients including the elderly with a treatment window of 6 hours from stroke onset, was seen as positive based on some post hoc analysis.

Thrombolysis slowly evolved to become a "standard of care" enthusiastically endorsed in guidelines by professional societies. Due to the questionable nature of benefit, a large number of practitioners however, remain skeptical and feel the advantage has been selectively highlighted and that there is a clear conflict of interest and point out that all the studies have been financed by industry.[13,14] These questions are justified, as the results are far from unequivocal. For example, in the latest IST-3 trial, one notes that the primary endpoint (proportion of patients who were alive and independent at 6 months) was similar in both groups. One also notes that there were more fatal and non-fatal intracranial hemorrhages and overall mortality in the thrombolysis group in the first 7 days, though the mortality subsequently became similar at 6 months. Despite that, this is viewed as a positive trial as some "benefit" was noted in a post hoc adjusted ordinal analysis, where at 6 months, more of the t-PA group had a favorable shift in functional score. Regardless, there seemed to be a concession that the benefit was marginal and something more needed to be done. This something was neuro-intervention, delivering the thrombolytic agent or a device to the culprit vessel and thereby restoring flow. In 1999, the first trial of intervention showed some questionable benefit.[15] A second trial in 2009 was essentially negative.[16] Later 3 trials in 2013 failed to show any meaningful benefit[17–19] and after a further period of refining the patient selection, the equipment and the technique, 5 trials in 2014-15 have shown benefit.[20–24]

In ARDS, four RCTs between 2001 and 2009 evaluated the effect of prone position and showed an improvement in oxygenation without a mortality benefit.[25–28] A 2010 meta-analysis of these RCTs suggested a mortality benefit in those with severe ARDS.[29] Finally, in 2013, an RCT in severe ARDS showed a mortality benefit.[30]

When a previously negative RCT for a specific therapy is followed by positive RCTs, it usually implies that the patient selection and the delivery of the treatment have been refined over a period of time. The learning curve of the therapy has been overcome, and the exact cohort which benefit have been identified. So, it is a good idea not to completely reject an ICU technique based on one or two trials. As an example, two recent High Frequency Oscillation Ventilation (HFOV) trials[31,32] have been negative in adult acute respiratory distress syndrome

Therapies like prone position ventilation in ARDS and neuro-intervention in stroke have evolved over many RCTs before a successful protocol & technique was identified.

(ARDS) patients, but it is likely that a future trial will demonstrate a better way of using the technique and the patient selection will be better focused on those who will benefit. Obviously, with negative trials in HFOV, it should not be used as a default in ARDS patients now, but careful selection of some patients may still have a role. Otherwise, its use should be limited to patients recruited in future trials.

A legitimate question is, does the implementation of EBM lead to better outcomes. One would presume so, but this is not yet well demonstrated. No study showed that in an ICU that consistently practiced EBM based therapies had better clinical outcomes than those that mixed EBM and clinical experience and expertise. Part of the problem is that EBM is based on degrees of certainty and there is also a lot of junk literature purporting to be EBM. So, it is worthwhile for a clinician to have the skills to read papers, including RCTs, and meta-analysis and gauge the value of each, rather than blindly going by the abstract and the conclusion. This will be explored in more detail in the section on protocols and guidelines and in the appendix on EBM.

Another aspect of EBM which needs clarification is that "lack of proof is not proof of lack". This means that if a specific aspect of therapy is not studied adequately, it is not automatically assumed to be ineffective. In hemodynamics, many aspects of monitoring are poorly studied. All the newer cardiac output monitoring devices have been minimally studied, usually by comparing it against another cardiac output monitor, rather than a clinical outcome. There is no useful evidence which can guide us as to when we should switch from fluids to vasoactive agents when trying to reverse hypotension. It is currently assumed that in early resuscitation a liberal fluid strategy is appropriate, but in prolonged resuscitation a more restrictive one is preferable. As of now, there are no RCTs which look at alternate resuscitation strategies for early versus prolonged resuscitation.

Unfortunately, the literature is vast and it helps to select useful literature, rather than be aware of all literature, a practically impossible task. We attempt to do so by selecting the following. First we look at literature of mainstream ICU therapies, such as hemodynamic management, mechanical ventilation in respiratory failure and renal replacement therapy (RRT) in renal failure. Then we focus on papers of therapies that achieved physiological or surrogate targets and yet harmed patients, highlighting the need to focus on clinical rather

One would presume that the implementation of EBM lead to better outcomes. But this is not yet demonstrated in clinical trials.

than surrogate end points. Then we look at literature that focuses on doing less rather than more in ICU as a possible way of improving outcomes.

As a starting point, we have listed all the RCTs in critical care and acute medicine which are from the New England Journal of Medicine (NEJM) in the last 8 years. These focus on mortality and clinical endpoints (Table 1 and 2) and we make some observations. This is not a cherry picked list (reader feedback is requested if we may have inadvertently missed any). It represents a selection of the better and more robust trials in the field of critical care, acute medicine and surgery. One could say they passed the NEJM peer review test and were selected by the editors to be the ones of most clinical interest to the general medical fraternity. They are all RCTs and nearly all focus on mortality, the most relevant clinical endpoint. They are divided into three categories: those that improved clinical outcomes, those that did not affect clinical outcomes and those that worsened clinical outcomes. The neutral ones predominate. In the successful ones, 5 out of 10 cover a single therapy, Endovascular Treatment for Stroke. The most obvious interpretation of this is that clinicians and academicians are not yet good enough in guessing as to which therapies will improve outcomes. This further implies that our understanding of pathophysiology, pharmacology and therapeutics is more superficial than we would like to believe. When subject to the test of improving clinical outcomes, the vast majority of our studies have been negative. Hopefully, as our understanding of physiology improves, we will be able to more accurately guess which therapies are going to improve clinical outcomes.

Pitfall No. 3

Following eminence based medicine rather than evidence based medicine for standard life sustaining ICU therapies.

In science, evidence means everything, authority means nothing. The largest amount of scientific eminence cannot trump the smallest amount of scientific evidence.

*– **Paul Lutus***

Pitfall No. 4

Chasing the wrong therapeutic target. Chasing a physiological or surrogate outcome rather than a clinical one.

"The Operation was successful but the patient died"

NEJM RCTs in Critical Care, Acute Medicine and Surgery

Table 1. ICU conditions			
Acute Respiratory Distress Syndrome	Statins in ARDS	NEGATIVE/NEUTRAL	*N Engl J Med* 2014;371:1695–703
	NMB in ARDS (ACURASYS)	POSITIVE	*N Engl J Med* 2010;363:1107–16
	Prone in Severe ARDS (PROSEVA)	POSITIVE	*N Engl J Med* 2013;368:2159–68
Renal failure/ Renal replacement Therapy	RRT Intensity: (VA/NIH ATN Trial)	NEGATIVE/NEUTRAL	*N Engl J Med.* 2008 Jul 3;359(1):7–20
	RRT Intensity: (RENAL Trial)	NEGATIVE/NEUTRAL	*N Engl J Med.* 2009 Oct 22;361(17):1627–38
	RRT/UF in cardiac failure	ADVERSE	*N Engl J Med* 2012; 367:2296–304
Shock and Sepsis	Albumin in Septic Shock (ALBIOS)	NEGATIVE/NEUTRAL	*N Engl J Med* 2014; 370:1412–21
	IABP in Cardiogenic shock	NEGATIVE/NEUTRAL	*N Engl J Med* 2012;367:1287–96
	Vasopressin vs. Noradrenaline (VASTT)	NEGATIVE/NEUTRAL	*N Engl J Med* 2008;358:877–87
	APC (PROWESS-SHOCK).	NEGATIVE/NEUTRAL	*N Engl J Med* 2012;366:2055
	Dopamine vs. Noradrenaline (SOAP)	NEGATIVE/NEUTRAL	*N Engl J Med* 2010;362:779–89
	BP Target (SEPSISPAM)	NEGATIVE/NEUTRAL	*N Engl J Med* 2014; 370:1583–93
	Steroids in Sepsis (CORTICUS)	NEGATIVE/NEUTRAL	*N Engl J Med* 2008;358:111–24
Fluids and Blood	HES (6S)	ADVERSE	*N Engl J Med* 2012;367:124–34
	HES (CHEST)	ADVERSE	*N Engl J Med* 2012;367:1901–11
	Fluid Bolus in Severe Infection (FEAST)	ADVERSE	*N Engl J Med* 2011;364:2483–95
	Liberal PRBC (TRISS)	NEGATIVE/NEUTRAL	*N Engl J Med* 2014;371:1381–91
	PRBC, old vs. fresh (ABLE)	NEGATIVE/NEUTRAL	*N Engl J Med* 2015;372:1410–18
Nutrition	Early TPN vs. EN (CALORIES)	NEGATIVE/NEUTRAL	*N Engl J Med* 2014;371:1673–84
	Glutamine	ADVERSE	*N Engl J Med* 2013;368:1489–97
	Early TPN	ADVERSE	*N Engl J Med* 2011;365:506–17
Ventilation	HFOV (OSCAR)	NEGATIVE/NEUTRAL	*N Engl J Med* 2013;368:806
	HFOV (OSCILLATE)	ADVERSE	*N Engl J Med* 2013;368:795–805
Blood Sugar	Tight Sugar Control (NICE- SUGAR)	ADVERSE	*N Engl J Med* 2009;360:1283–97

Table 2. Medical and surgical conditions			
Condition	**Therapy**	**Outcome**	**Reference**
Stroke	Thrombolysis in stroke (ECASS III)	POSITIVE	*N Engl J Med* 2008;359:1317–29
	Hemi Craniotomy for MCA Infarct in Elderly (DESTINY II)	POSITIVE	*N Engl J Med* 2014;370:1091–1100
	Endovascular Treatment for Stroke (MR CLEAN)	POSITIVE	*N Engl J Med* 2015;372:11–20.
	Endovascular Treatment for Stroke. (EXTEND-IA)	POSITIVE	*N Engl J Med* 2015;372:1009–18.
	Endovascular Treatment for Stroke (ESCAPE)	POSITIVE	*N Engl J Med* 2015;372:1019–30.
	Endovascular Treatment for Stroke (SWIFT PRIME)	POSITIVE	*N Engl J Med* 2015;372:2285–95.
	Endovascular Treatment for Stroke (REVASCAT)	POSITIVE	*N Engl J Med* 2015;372:2296–306.
	Endovascular Treatment for Stroke (MR RESCUE)	NEGATIVE/NEUTRAL	*N Engl J Med* 2013;368:914–23
	Endovascular Treatment for Stroke (SYNTHESIS)	NEGATIVE/NEUTRAL	*N Engl J Med* 2013;368:904–13.
	Endovascular Treatment for Stroke (IMS III)	NEGATIVE/NEUTRAL	*N Engl J Med* 2013;368:893–903.
	BP control in ICH (INTERACT 2)	NEGATIVE/NEUTRAL	*N Engl J Med* 2013; 368:2355–65
Traumatic Brain Injury	Progesterone in TBI (PROTECT III)	NEGATIVE/NEUTRAL	*N Engl J Med* 2014; 371:2457–66
	Progesterone in TBI (SYNAPSE)	NEGATIVE/NEUTRAL	*N Engl J Med* 2014; 371:2467–76
	ICP monitoring	NEGATIVE/NEUTRAL	*N Engl J Med* 2012;367:2471–81
	Surgical ICP control (DECRA)	ADVERSE	*N Engl J Med* 2011; 364:1493–1502
Resuscitation	Hypothermia Post CPR (TTM)	NEGATIVE/NEUTRAL	*N Engl J Med* 2013; 369:2197–2206
	Hypothermia Post CPR Pediatrics (THAPCA)	NEGATIVE/NEUTRAL	*N Engl J Med* 2015;372:1898–908
Pulmonary Embolism and Deep Vein Thrombosis	LMWH vs. UFH (PROTECT).	NEGATIVE/NEUTRAL	*N Engl J Med* 2011; 364:1305–14
	LMWH DVT Prophylaxis (LIFENOX).	NEGATIVE/NEUTRAL	*N Engl J Med* 2011; 365:2463–72
	Thrombolysis in PE (PEITHO)	NEGATIVE/NEUTRAL	*N Engl J Med* 2014; 370:1402–11
Early Goal Directed Therapy	EGDT (ProCESS)	NEGATIVE/NEUTRAL	*N Engl J Med* 2014; 370:1683–93
	EGDT (ARISE)	NEGATIVE/NEUTRAL	*N Engl J Med* 2014; 371:1496–1506
	EGDT (ProMISe)	NEGATIVE/NEUTRAL	*N Engl J Med* 2015; 372:1301–11
Pancreatitis	Minimally Invasive Approach in Pancreatitis	POSITIVE	*N Engl J Med* 2010;362:1491–1502.
Selective Digestive Decontamination	Decontamination of the Digestive Tract and Oropharynx	NEUTRAL (Positive after data adjustment)	*N Engl J Med* 2009;360:20–31.

Pitfall No. 5

Doing too much. Choosing a liberal approach of using all possible treatments, instead of a restrictive approach of judiciously using proven or highly plausible treatments.

The best practitioners give to their patients the least medicine.

– Frederick Saunders

References

1. Emanuel Rivers, Ryant Nguyen, Uzanne Havstad *et al.* Early goal-directed therapy in the treatment of severe sepsis and septic shock. *N Engl J Med* 2001;345:1368–77.
2. Jansen TC, van Bommel J, Schoonderbeek FJ, *et al.* for the LACTATE study group. Early Lactate-Guided Therapy in Intensive Care Unit Patients. A Multicenter, Open-Label, Randomized Controlled Trial. *Am J Respir Crit Care Med* 2010;182:752–61.
3. ProMISe Trial Investigators. Trial of Early, Goal-Directed Resuscitation for Septic Shock. *N Engl J Med* 2015;372:1301–11.
4. The ARISE Investigators and the ANZICS Clinical Trials Group. Goal-Directed Resuscitation for Patients with Early Septic Shock. *N Engl J Med* 2014;371:1496–506.
5. The ProCESS Investigators a Randomized Trial of Protocol-Based Care for Early Septic Shock. *N Engl J Med* 2014;370:1683–93.
6. The National Institute of Neurological Disorders and Stroke rt-PA Stroke Study Group. Tissue plasminogen activator for acute ischemic stroke. *N Engl J Med* 1995;333:1581–88.
7. Kwiatkowski TG, Libman RB, Frankel M, *et al.* Effects of tissue plasminogen activator for acute ischemic stroke at one year. *N Engl J Med* 1999;340:1781–87.
8. Hacke W, Kaste M, Fieschi C, *et al.* Intravenous thrombolysis with recombinant tissue plasminogen activator for acute hemispheric stroke: the European Cooperative Acute Stroke Study (ECASS). *JAMA* 1995;274:1017–25.
9. Hacke W, Kaste M, Fieschi C, *et al.* Randomized double-blind placebo-controlled trial of thrombolytic therapy with intravenous alteplase in acute ischemic stroke (ECASS II). *Lancet* 1998;352:1245–51.
10. Hacke W, Kaste M, Bluhmki E, *et al.* Thrombolysis with alteplase 3 to 4.5 hours after acute ischemic stroke. ECASS III. *N Engl J Med* 2008;359:1317–29.
11. Clark WM, Wissman S, Albers GW, *et al.* Recombinant tissue-type plasminogen activator (alteplase) for ischemic stroke 3 to 5 hours after symptom onset: the ATLANTIS study: a randomized controlled trial. *JAMA* 1999;282:2019–26.
12. The IST-3 collaborative group. The benefits and harms of intravenous thrombolysis with recombinant tissue plasminogen activator within 6 h of acute ischemic stroke (the third international stroke trial [IST-3]): a randomized controlled trial. *Lancet* 2012;379:2352–63.
13. Jeanne Lenzer. Alteplase for stroke: money and optimistic claims buttress the "brain attack" campaign. *BMJ* 2002;324:723.
14. Jeanne Lenzer. Why we can't trust clinical guidelines. *BMJ* 2013;346:f3830.
15. Furlan A, Higashida R, Wechsler L, *et al.* Intra-arterial prourokinase for acute ischemic stroke — the PROACT II study: a randomized controlled trial. *JAMA* 1999;282:2003–11.

16. Mazighi M, Serfaty JM, Labreuche J, *et al.* Comparison of intravenous alteplase with a combined intravenous-endovascular approach in patients with stroke and confirmed arterial occlusion (RECANALISE study): a prospective cohort study. *Lancet Neurol* 2009;8:802–9.
17. Broderick JP, Palesch YY, Demchuk AM, *et al.* Endovascular therapy after intravenous t-PA versus t-PA alone for stroke. The IMS-3study: *N Engl J Med* 2013;368:893–903.
18. Kidwell CS, Jahan R, Gornbein J, *et al.* A trial of imaging selection and endovascular treatment for ischemic stroke. The MR RESCUE study: *N Engl J Med* 2013;368:914–23.
19. Ciccone A, Valvassori L, Nichelatti M, *et al.* Endovascular treatment for acute ischemic stroke. The SYNTHESIS Expansion study: *N Engl J Med* 2013;368:904–13.
20. Berkhemer OA, Fransen PSS, Beumer D, *et al.* A randomized trial of intra-arterial treatment for acute ischemic stroke. (MR CLEAN) *N Engl J Med* 2015;372:11–20.
21. Campbell BCV, Mitchell PJ, Kleinig TJ, *et al.* Endovascular therapy for ischemic stroke with perfusion-imaging selection. (EXTEND-IA) *N Engl J Med* 2015;372:1009–18.
22. Goyal M, Demchuk AM, Menon BK, *et al.* Randomized assessment of rapid endovascular treatment of ischemic stroke. (ESCAPE) *N Engl J Med* 2015;372:1019–30.
23. Saver JL, Goyal M, Bonafe A, *et al.* Stent-retriever thrombectomy after intravenous t-PA vs. t-PA alone in stroke. (SWIFT PRIME) *N Engl J Med* 2015;372:2285–95.
24. Jovin TG, Chamorro A, Cobo E, *et al.* Thrombectomy within 8 hours after symptom onset in ischemic stroke. (REVASCAT) *N Engl J Med* 2015;372:2296–306.
25. Gattinoni L, Tognoni G, Pesenti A, *et al*; Prone-Supine Study Group. Effect of prone positioning on the survival of patients with acute respiratory failure. *N Engl J Med* 2001;345:568–73.
26. Guerin C, Gaillard S, Lemasson S, *et al.* Effects of systematic prone positioning in hypoxemic acute respiratory failure: a randomized controlled trial. *JAMA* 2004;292:2379–87.
27. Mancebo J, Ferna´ ndez R, Blanch L, *et al.* A multicenter trial of prolonged prone ventilation in severe acute respiratory distress syndrome. *Am J Respir Crit Care Med* 2006;173:1233–39.
28. Taccone P, Pesenti A, Latini R, *et al*; Prone-Supine II Study Group. Prone positioning in patients with moderate and severe acute respiratory distress syndrome: a randomized controlled trial. *JAMA* 2009;302:1977–84.
29. Sud S, Friedrich JO, Taccone P, *et al.* Prone ventilation reduces mortality in patients with acute respiratory failure and severe hypoxemia: systematic review and meta-analysis. *Intensive Care Med* 2010;36:585–99.
30. Claude Guérin, Jean Reignier, Jean-Christophe Richard, *et al.* for the PROSEVA Study Group. Prone Positioning in Severe Acute Respiratory Distress Syndrome. *N Engl J Med* 2013;368:2159–68.
31. Ferguson ND, Cook DJ, Guyatt GH, *et al.* High-frequency oscillation in early acute respiratory distress syndrome. *N Engl J Med* 2013;368:795–805.
32. Young D, Lamb SE, Shah S,*et al.* High-frequency oscillation for acute respiratory distress syndrome. *N Engl J Med* 2013;368:806–13.

Pitfall No. 3

Eminence vs Evidence Based Medicine

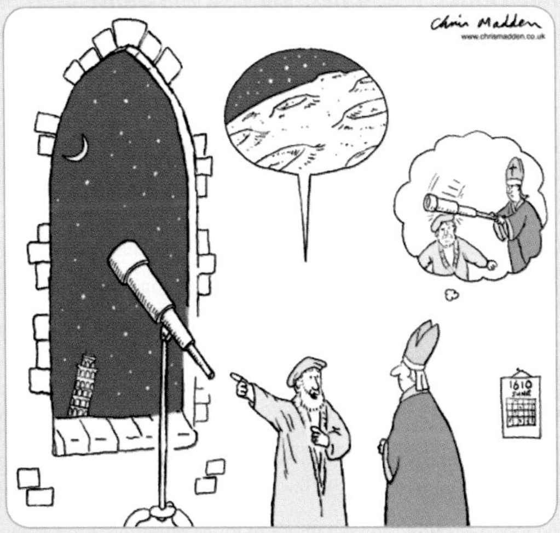

> "A little misunderstanding?!
>
> **Galileo & the Pope** had a little misunderstanding."
>
> Dr. Sheldon Cooper

Pitfall No. 3

Eminence Based Medicine Instead of Evidence Based Medicine for Standard ICU Therapies

"Eminence Based Medicine: Making the same mistakes with increasing confidence over an impressive number of years"

– O'Donnell M. (from A Sceptic's Medical Dictionary).

Review of Literature

The earlier chapter reviewed some aspects of evidence based medicine (EBM) relevant to critical care. In this chapter, we specifically focus on the newer and more robust trials that evaluate major topics and therapies in critical care. The selection focuses on large randomized control trials (RCTs) with clinically meaningful endpoints, preferably mortality. These trials cover the standard treatments used in the intensive care unit (ICU) that include management of shock and hemodynamic monitoring, mechanical ventilation, renal failure and renal replacement therapy. For each topic, we first briefly cover current concepts, we then look at the evidence to evaluate how many of these concepts are scientifically valid, and we lastly summarize our pragmatic take home messages from these studies.

Shock and Hemodynamics

Theoretical and Pathophysiological Considerations

Conventional thinking in hemodynamics and shock go something like this. The plan is to target a mean blood pressure above 65 mmHg as that is the point auto-regulation fails. One needs to ensure that the arterial pressure is achieving perfusion, that can be evaluated by the warmth of the extremities, the mentation and the urine output. The arterial or venous lactate partly reflect perfusion, and falling lactate levels are usually a marker of successful resuscitation. In order to achieve this target, the simplest option is to fill the circulation using the CVP as a guide. More "advanced" monitoring of cardiac output, using either a pulmonary artery catheter or one of the many newer devices such as FloTrac, LIDCO or PICCO, allow one to fine tune the management. Then looking specifically at certain parameters like the mixed pulmonary artery (SvO_2) or superior vena cava oxygen ($ScvO_2$) saturation and also calculating the systemic oxygen delivery and consumption will help. One can evaluate more dynamic parameters like stroke volume variation or pulse pressure variation or passive leg raising test that can be used to further evaluate fluid responsiveness. If the patient is fluid responsive, they should be given more fluids. Colloids and albumin leak less from the circulation and are therefore preferable. If this does not restore the pressure and the perfusion, one should then add an inotrope to improve the cardiac output. This usually involves choosing a catecholamine with beta stimulating properties. If this too does not improve the BP, a vasopressor such as noradrenaline should be added. Although, the above plan sounds reasonable a series of recent trials have made us question the validity of this strictly physiological approach.

Evidence

There have been a large number of well-conducted RCTs looking at clinical endpoints on this subject in the last 5–10 years. Review of recent trials include those which look at BP targets, choice of fluids, choice of vasoactive drugs and early goal directed therapy. We finally look at a couple of studies that have thrown some surprising results.

Blood Pressure Targets

Based on animal studies and human physiological studies, the Mean Arterial Pressure (MAP) of 65 mmHg is accepted as the standard target for patients with septic shock.[1] To date, in the context of the ICU patient, no studies have evaluated MAP targets less than 65 mm Hg. Recently a large study (SEPSISPAM) has compared a higher target and the investigators concluded that targeting a mean arterial pressure of 80 to 85 mm Hg, as compared with 65 to 70 mmHg, among patients with septic shock undergoing resuscitation did not result in significant differences in mortality at either 28 or 90 days.[2] They did note less renal injury and need for renal replacement therapy (RRT) with high mean blood pressure (MBP) in previously hypertensive patients, and they also noted more atrial fibrillation (AF) in high MBP group (see Figures 1-2 and Table 1 from paper).

Another very large observational trial looked at blood pressure *intra-operatively* in 33,300 patients[3] and noted that even short durations of an intra-operative MAP less than 55 mmHg are associated with acute kidney injury (AKI) and myocardial injury. The longer the blood pressure (BP) stayed less than 55 mmHg, the more the renal and cardiac injury.

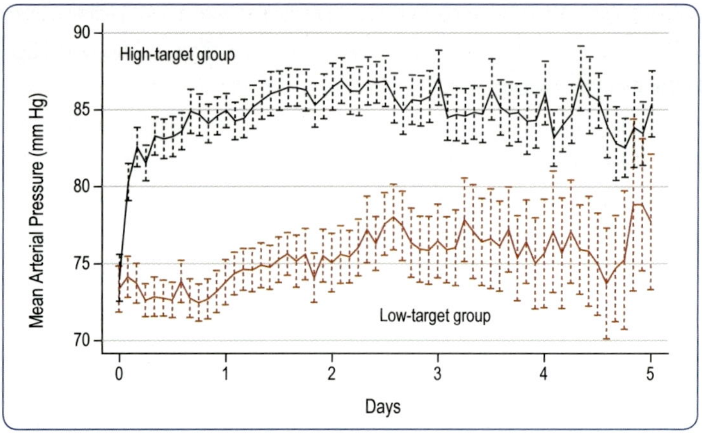

Figure 1. SEPSISPAM Blood pressure achieved in both groups[2]

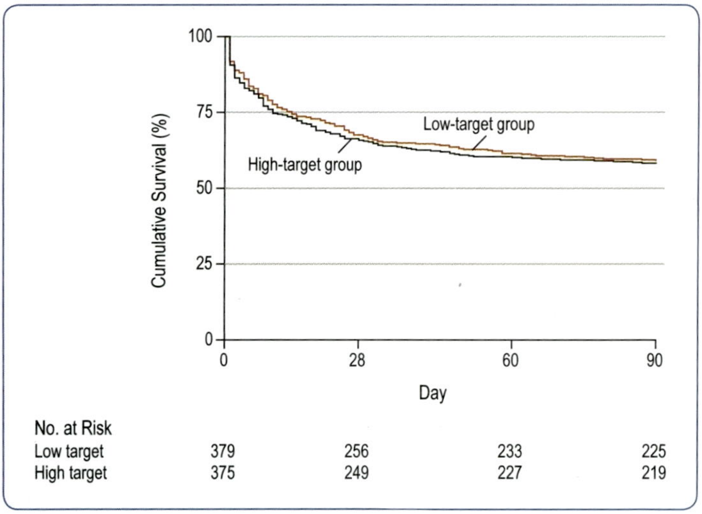

Figure 2. SEPSISPAM Mortality in each group[2]

The target BP for the bleeding trauma patient is not so straight forward. Here any low BP that maintains perfusion is acceptable till the bleeding has been surgically corrected. Two trials compared "hypotensive resuscitation" during active hemorrhage. One compared a target SBP of 70 vs 100 mmHg,[4] while the other compared a target MBP of 50 vs 65 mmHg.[5] In both the studies, the outcomes were the same but there was less transfusion requirements in those with lower targeted pressure.

Table 1. SEPSISPAM Outcomes and Adverse Events in each group[2]

Variable	Low-Target Group (*N* = 388)	High-Target Group (*N* = 388)	P Value
Cumulative fluid intake from day 1 to day 5 — liters	10.0 (5.8–14.0)	10.5 (5.5–14.0)	0.89
Cumulative urine output from day 1 to day 5 — liters	6.7 (2.9–10.7)	6.9 (2.4–10.7)	0.87
Cumulative fluid balance from day 1 to day 5 — liters	2.8 (0.0–6.2)	2.4 (0.0–6.0)	0.74
Median dose of norepinephrine (IQR) — μg/kg/min			
Day 1	0.45 (0.17–1.21)	0.58 (0.26–1.80)	<0.001
Day 2	0.16 (0.03–0.48)	0.38 (0.14–0.90)	<0.001
Day 3	0.02 (0.00–0.16)	0.14 (0.01–0.50)	<0.001
Day 4	0.00 (0.00–0.05)	0.03 (0.00–0.22)	<0.001
Day 5	0.00 (0.00–0.03)	0.01 (0.00–0.15)	<0.001
Duration of catecholamine infusion — days	3.7±3.2	4.7±3.7	<0.001
Primary outcome: death at day 28 — no. (%)*	132 (34.0)	142 (36.6)	0.57
Secondary outcomes — no./total no. (%)			
Death at day 90†	164 (42.3)	170 (43.8)	0.74
Survival at day 28 without organ support‡	241 (62.1)	235 (60.6)	0.66
Doubling of plasma creatinine	161 (41.5)	150 (38.7)	0.42
No chronic hypertension	71/215 (33.0)	85/221 (38.5)	0.32
Chronic hypertension	90/173 (52.0)	65/167 (38.9)	0.02
Renal-replacement therapy from day 1 to day 7	139 (35.8)	130 (33.5)	0.50
No chronic hypertension	66/215 (30.7)	77/221 (34.8)	0.36
Chronic hypertension	73/173 (42.2)	53/167 (31.7)	0.046
Serious adverse events — no. (%)			
Any	69 (17.8)	74 (19.1)	0.64
Acute myocardial infarction§	2 (0.5)	7 (1.8)	0.18
Atrial fibrillation	11 (2.8)	26 (6.7)	0.02
Ventricular fibrillation or tachycardia	15 (3.9)	22 (5.7)	0.24
Digital ischemia	9 (2.3)	10 (2.6)	0.82
Mesenteric ischemia	9 (2.3)	9 (2.3)	1.00
Bleeding	42 (10.8)	31 (8.0)	0.22

Bottom Lines:

- When following a pressure target, ensure that perfusion is maintained at that target.
- In septic shock target MBP of > 65 mmHg, except in previously hypertensive patients in whom target >80-85 mmHg.

- Intra-operatively, prevent even brief periods of hypotension by avoiding MBP of less than 55 mmHg.
- In exsanguinating trauma, accept low systolic blood pressure (SBP) of 70 or mean arterial blood pressure (MBP) of 50 mmHg till the bleeding has been surgically controlled.

Choice of Fluids

There have been innumerable debates and controversies about the choice of fluids, specifically crystalloids versus colloids and also between albumin, saline, "balanced fluids" and chloride poor fluids. The discussion below is based on 5 recent RCTs discussing the benefits of the various fluid choices. One of the first good studies addressing this debate, was the SAFE study[6] which demonstrated that saline and albumin in saline were equivalent as resuscitation fluids. Then came the starch versus saline studies which were all published in the same year 2012, but were conducted in 3 different continents, CRYSTMAS in the US, 6S in Scandinavia and CHEST in Australia.

The relatively small CRYSTMAS study,[7] showed that early hemodynamic stability could be achieved among patients with septic shock using a significantly smaller volume of Hydroxyethyl Starch (HES) than of sodium chloride (NaCl). At the same time, HES did not appear to be associated with any increase in adverse events.

The large 6S trial,[8] showed that patients with severe sepsis assigned to fluid resuscitation with HES 130/0.4 had an increased risk of death at day 90 and were more likely to require renal replacement therapy, as compared with those receiving Ringer's acetate. The mortality and other outcomes are shown in Figure 3 and Table 2 below.

The other large trial CHEST,[9] showed that among patients in the ICU, there was no significant difference in 90 day mortality between patients resuscitated with 6% HES (130/0.4) or saline. However, more patients who received resuscitation with HES were treated with renal replacement therapy. The mortality and other outcomes are shown in Figure 4 and Table 3 below.

The CRISTAL trial[10] was a more pragmatic trial and showed an opposite effect. Among ICU patients with hypovolemia, the use of colloids versus crystalloids did not result in a significant difference in their chosen primary end point, 28 day mortality. A secondary endpoint, the 90 day mortality was lower among patients receiving colloids. The mortality is shown below in Figure 5.

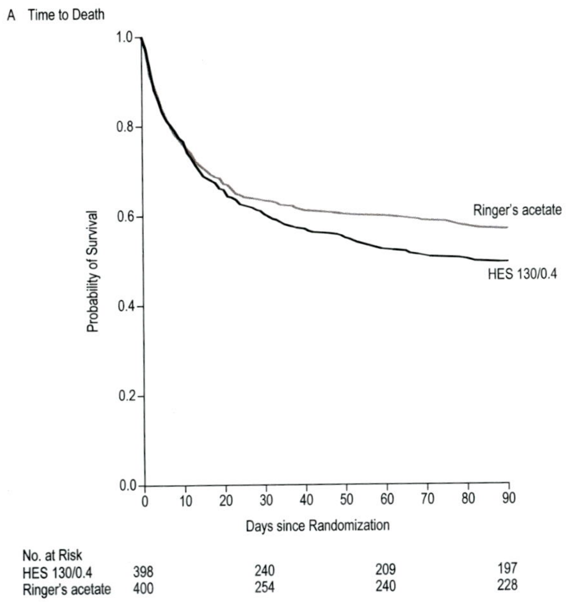

Figure 3. 6S trial. Mortality in each group[8]

Table 2. 6S trial. Primary and Secondary Outcomes[2]

Outcome	HES 130/0.42 (N = 398)	Ringer's Acetate (N = 400)	Relative Risk (95% CI)	P Value
Primary outcome				
Dead or dependent on dialysis at day 90 — no. (%)	202 (51)	173 (43)	1.17 (1.01–1.36)	0.03
Dead at day 90 — no. (%)	201 (51)	172 (43)	1.17 (1.01–1.36)	0.03
Dependent on dialysis at day 90 — no. (%)	1 (0.25)	1 (0.25)	—	1.00
Secondary outcome measures				
Dead at day 28 — no. (%)	154 (39)	144 (36)	1.08 (0.90–1.28)	0.43
Severe bleeding — no. (%)†	38 (10)	25 (6)	1.52 (0.94–2.48)	0.09
Severe allergic reaction — no. (%)†	1 (0.25)	0	—	0.32
SOFA score at day 5 — median (interquartile range)	6 (2–11)	6 (0–10)	—	0.64
Use of renal-replacement therapy — no. (%)‡	87 (22)	65 (16)	1.35 (1.01–1.80)	0.04
Use of renal-replacement therapy or renal SOFA score ≥3 — no. (%)§	129 (32)	108 (27)	1.20 (0.97–1.48)	0.10
Doubling of plasma creatinine level — no. (%)†	148 (41)	127 (35)	1.18 (0.98–1.43)	0.08
Acidosis — no. (%)†¶	307 (77)	312 (78)	0.99 (0.92–1.06)	0.72
Alive without renal-replacement therapy — mean % of days ‖	91	93	—	0.048

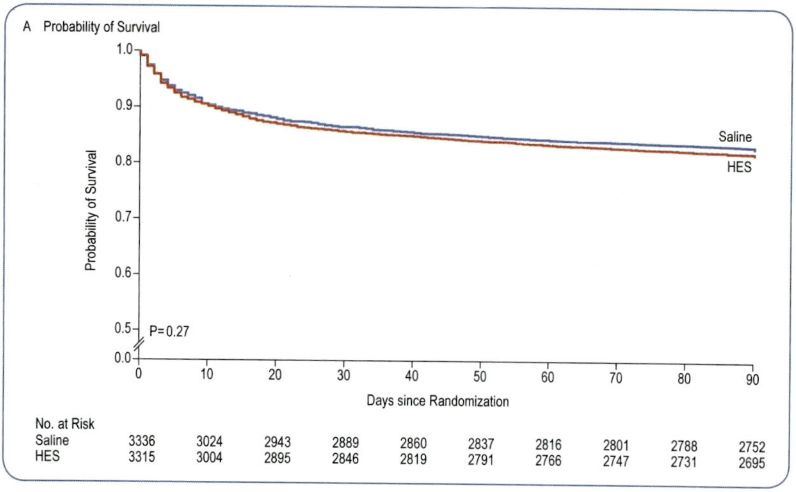

Figure 4. CHEST Mortality[9]

Table 3. CHEST Outcomes and Adverse Events[9]

Variable	HES	Saline	Relative Risk (95% CI)	P Value
Outcome				
Primary outcome of death at day 90 — no./total no. (%)	597/3315 (18.0)	566/3336 (17.0)	1.06 (0.96 to 1.18)	0.26
Secondary outcomes — no./total no. (%)				
Renal outcomes				
RIFLE-R	1788/3309 (54.0)	1912/3335 (57.3)	0.94 (0.90 to 0.98)	0.007
RIFLE-I	1130/3265 (34.6)	1253/3300 (38.0)	0.91 (0.85 to 0.97)	0.005
RIFLE-F	336/3243 (10.4)	301/3263 (9.2)	1.12 (0.97 to 1.30)	0.12
Use of renal-replacement therapy	235/3352 (7.0)	196/3375 (5.8)	1.21 (1.00 to 1.45)	0.04
New organ failure†				
Respiratory	540/2062 (26.2)	524/2094 (25.0)	1.05 (0.94 to 1.16)	0.39
Cardiovascular	663/1815 (36.5)	722/1808 (39.9)	0.91 (0.84 to 0.99)	0.03
Coagulation	142/2987 (4.8)	119/3010 (4.0)	1.20 (0.95 to 1.53)	0.13
Hepatic	55/2830 (1.9)	36/2887 (1.2)	1.56 (1.03 to 2.36)	0.03
Tertiary outcomes — no./total no. (%)				
Death in ICU	364/3313 (11.0)	360/3331 (10.8)	1.02 (0.89 to 1.17)	0.81

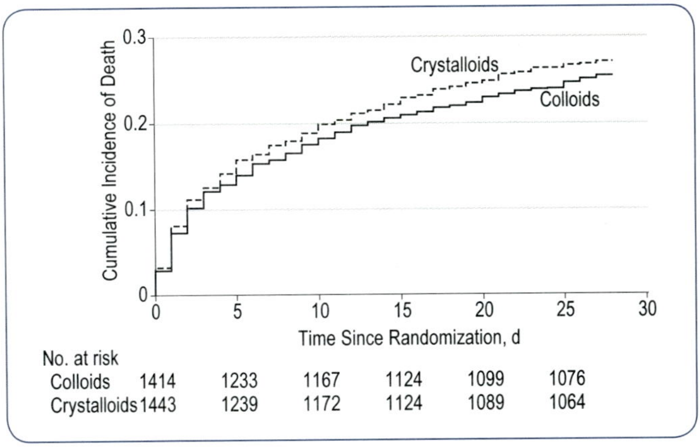

Figure 5. CRISTAL trial. Mortality[10]

Lastly, the ALBIOS trial[11] in 2014 used albumin to correct a low albumin among patients who were already adequately volume resuscitated. They concluded that among patients with severe sepsis, albumin replacement to correct hypoalbuminemia in addition to crystalloids, as compared with crystalloids alone, did not improve the rate of survival at 28 and 90 days. The mortality is shown below in Figure 6.

But then a meta-analysis of large albumin RCTs showed a mortality benefit (Figure 7).[12]

It is difficult to get a single message out of these (and some subsequent subgroup and meta-analysis). Some possible take home messages are:

- In general crystalloids and colloids are associated with similar outcomes.
- The use of starch solutions may be deleterious among patients with renal injury or with the more severe forms of sepsis and they should be avoided in these patients.
- Routine replacement of albumin is not useful, but some subgroup analysis and a meta-analysis suggest that it might be beneficial in severe sepsis.

Choice of Vasoactive Agents

Conventionally vasoactive agents were viewed as being inotropes or vasoconstrictors, and the choice depended on whether the patient was in a low flow state or a vasodilated state. In sepsis and in any long standing form of shock, both components may be present. Four trials have compared these agents and found little difference in outcomes.

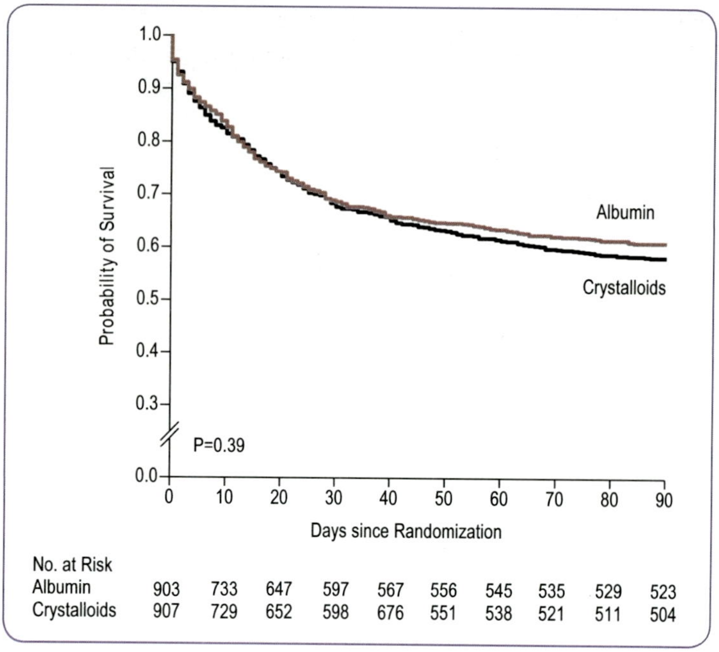

Figure 6. ALBIOS trial. Mortality[11]

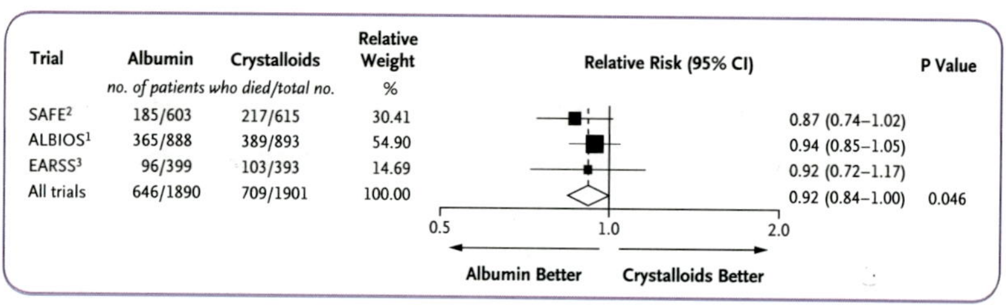

Figure 7. Meta Analysis of Albumin RCTs[12]

Of the four, the first looked at noradrenaline plus dobutamine versus adrenaline alone[13] and demonstrated that there is no evidence of a difference in mortality and safety between adrenaline alone and noradrenaline plus dobutamine for the management of septic shock (Table 4 and Figure 8 below).

The second similarly compared adrenaline and noradrenaline[14] and found no difference in the achievement of a MAP goal and in mortality between adrenaline and noradrenaline in a

Table 4. Mortality in Adrenaline vs Noradrenaline + Dobutamine Trial[13]			
	Epinephrine (N = 161)	Norepinephrine plus dobutamine (N = 169)	P
At day 7	40 (25%)	34 (20%)	0.30
At day 14	56 (35%)	44 (26%)	0.08
At day 28	64 (40%)	58 (34%)	0.31
At discharge from intensive care	75 (47%)	75 (44%)	0.69
At discharge from hospital	84 (52%)	82 (49%)	0.51
At day 90	84 (52%)	85 (50%)	0.73

Data are number of details (%).

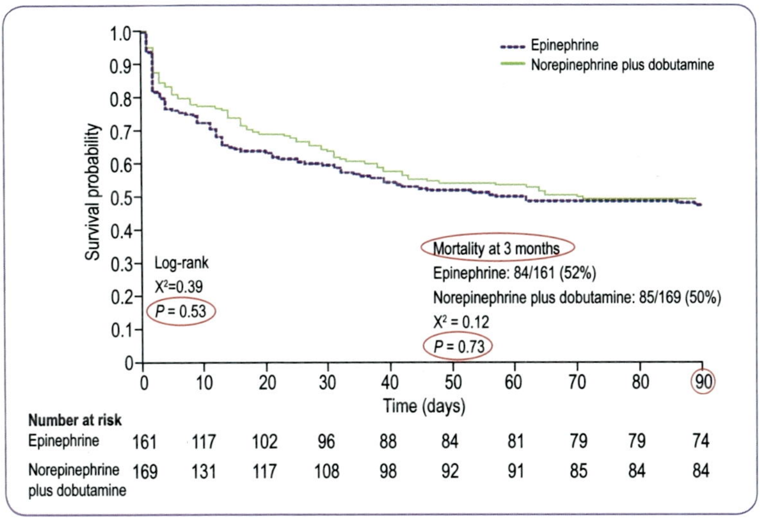

Figure 8. Mortality in Adrenaline vs. noradrenaline + Dobutamine Trial[13]

heterogeneous population of ICU patients (Table 5). They did note that the adrenaline group had a transient early hyperlactatemia and tachycardia (Figure 9 and 10), though this did not adversely impact outcome.

A trial comparing dopamine and noradrenaline[15] showed that there was no significant difference in the rate of death between patients with shock who were treated with dopamine as the first-line vasopressor agent and those who were treated with noradrenaline (Figure 11). They noted that the use of dopamine was associated with a greater number of adverse

Table 5. Mortality in Adrenaline vs Noradrenaline Trial[14]

Variables	Epinephrine	Norepinephrine	Hazard ratio	95% CI	P
All patients					
Time to achievement of MAP goal (h)	35.1 (13.8–70.4)	40.0 (14.5–120)	0.88	0.69–1.12	0.26
Day 28 mortality	31/138 (22.5)	36/138 (26.1)	0.86	0.57–1.31	0.48
Day 90 mortality	41/135 (30.4)	46/134 (34.3)	0.88	0.63–1.25	0.49
Patients with severe sepsis					
Time to achievement of MAP goal (h)	35.1 (16.7–75)	50.5 (18.2–127)	0.81	0.59–1.12	0.18
Day 28 mortality	17/76 (22.4)	24/82 (29.3)	0.76	0.45–1.31	0.32
Day 90 mortality	23/74 (31.1)	30/82 (36.6)	0.85	0.53–1.32	0.47
Patients with acute circulatory failure					
Time to achievement of MAP goal (h)	38.6 (18.0–85.7)	40.0 (15.1–122.8)	0.89	0.62–1.27	0.49
Day 28 mortality	15/64 (23.4)	17/63 (27.0)	0.87	0.48–1.58	0.65
Day 90 mortality	20/62 (32.3)	25/61 (41.0)	0.78	0.49–1.28	0.32

Time in hours expressed as median (interquartile range); mortality expressed as n/N (%); 95% CI = 95% confidence intervals

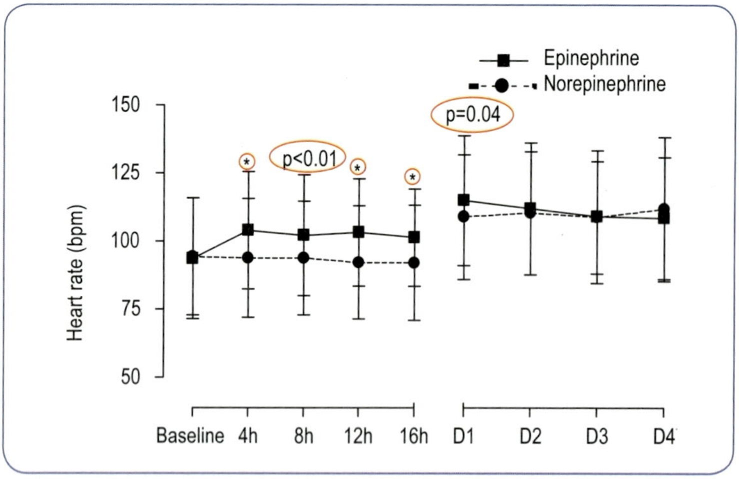

Figure 9. Heart Rate in Adrenaline vs Noradrenaline Trial[14]

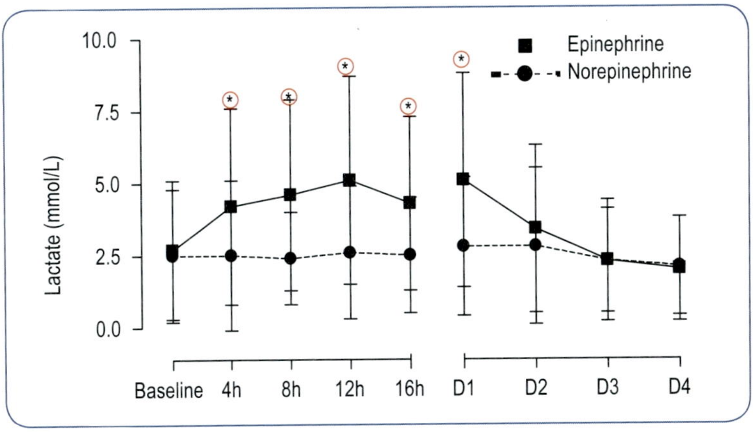

Figure 10. Lactate in Adrenaline vs. Noradrenaline Trial[14]

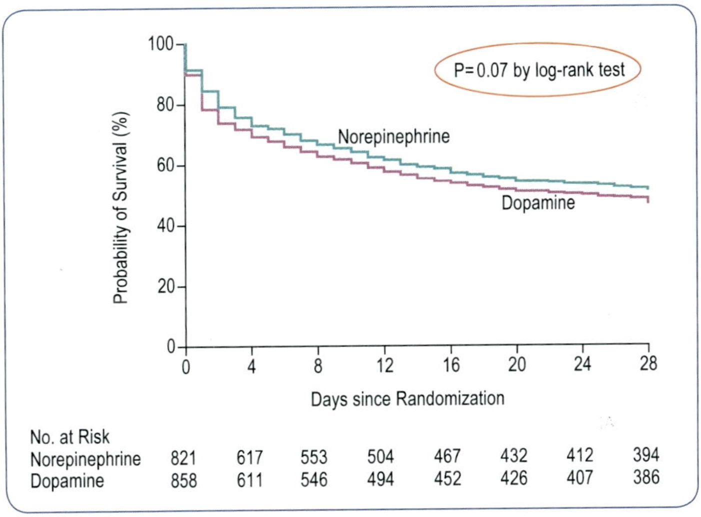

Figure 11. Mortality in Noradrenaline vs. Dopamine trial[15]

events and it caused more arrhythmias (Table 6). In a sub group analysis, they also noted that noradrenaline had better outcomes in cardiogenic shock (Figure 12).

A meta-analysis of 6 trials comparing dopamine and noradrenaline concluded that in septic shock, dopamine administration is associated with greater mortality and a higher incidence of arrhythmic events compared to noradrenaline administration (Figure 13).[16]

Table 6. Adverse effects in Noradrenaline vs. Dopamine trial[15]			
	Dopamine	Noradrenaline	
Arrhythmias — no. (%)	207 (24.1)	102 (12.4)	<0.001
Atrial fibrillation	176 (20.5)	90 (11.0)	
Ventricular tachycardia	21 (2.4)	8 (1.0)	
Ventricular fibrillation	10 (1.2)	4 (0.5)	
Myocardial infarction — no. (%)	19 (2.2)	25 (3.0)	0.29
New infectious episode			
No. of episodes			0.69
Median	1	1	
Interquartile range	0–1	0–1	
Patients with at least one episode — no. (%)	674 (78.6)	619 (75.4)	0.35
Skin ischemia — no. (%)	56 (6.5)	34 (4.1)	0.09
Mild†	46 (5.4)	28 (3.4)	
Severe‡	10 (1.2)	6 (0.7)	
Arterial occlusion — no. (%)§	23 (2.7)	20 (2.4)	0.12
Arms or fingers	5 (0.6)	1 (0.1)	
Legs	7 (0.8)	13 (1.6)	
Bowel	11 (1.3)	6 (0.7)	

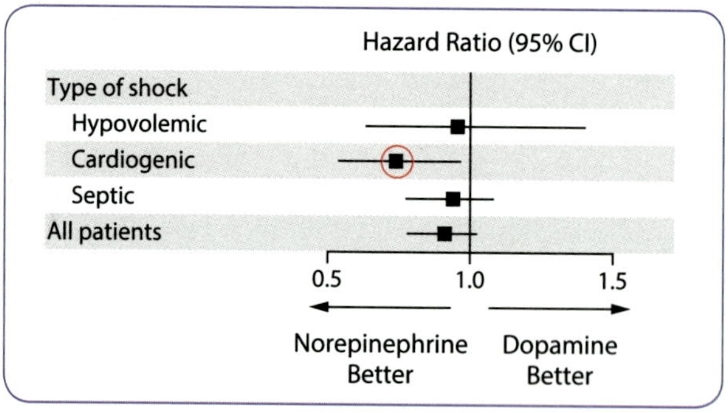

Figure 12. Subgroup outcomes in Noradrenaline vs. Dopamine trial[15]

The above three trials compared these agents as first line vasoactive drugs.

One trial looked at vasopressin versus noradrenaline[17] among patients with refractory shock who were not responding to standard doses of noradrenaline (Figure 14). They found that low-dose vasopressin did not reduce mortality rates as compared to high-dose

Study	Norepinephrine		Dopamine		
	Event	Total	Event	Total	RR [95% CI]
Martin *et al.*	7	16	10	16	1.43 [0.73–2.80]
Marilk *et al.*	5	10	6	10	1.20 [0.54–2.67]
Ruokonen *et al.*	4	5	3	5	0.75 [0.32–1.74]
Mathur *et al.*	14	25	19	25	1.36 [0.90–2.05]
De Backer *et al.*	249	502	291	542	1.08 [0.98–1.19]
Patel *et al.*	51	118	67	134	1.16 [0.89–1.51]
Overall	**330**	**676**	**396**	**732**	**1.12 [1.01–1.20]**

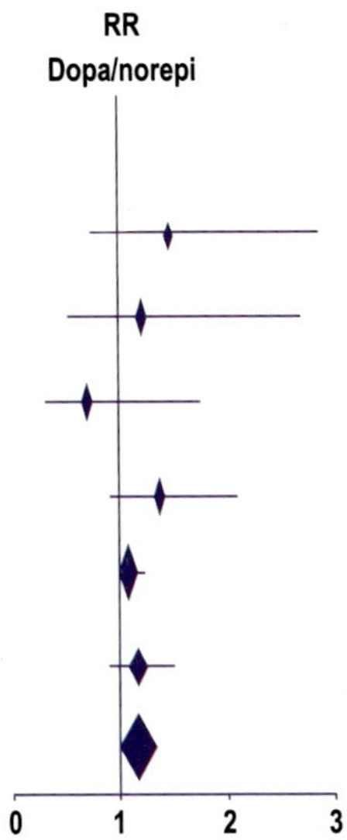

Figure 13. Meta analysis of Noradrenaline vs dopamine trials[16]

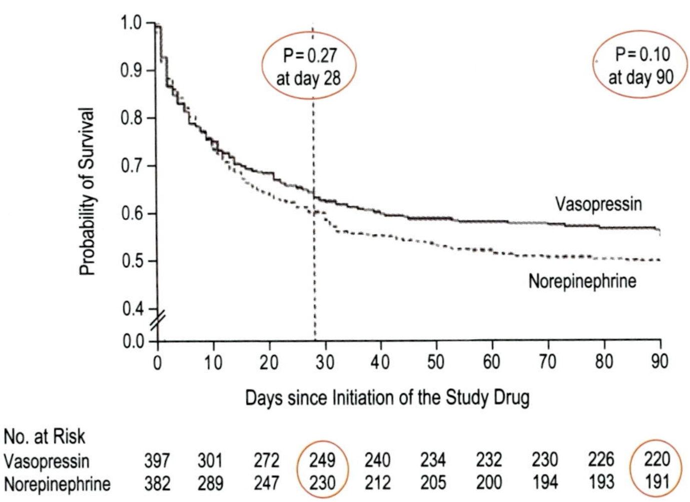

Figure 14. Mortality in Noradrenaline vs Vasopressin Trial [17]

Table 7. Subgroup outcomes in Noradrenaline vs Vasopressin Trial[17]

Stratum	Norepinephrine Group	Vasopressin Group	P Value†	Absolute Risk Reduction (95% CI)	Relative Risk (95% CI)
	no./total no. (%)			%	
More severe septic shock					
28-day mortality	85/200 (42.5)	88/200 (44.0)	0.76	−1.5 (−11.2 to 8.2)	1.04 (0.83 to 1.3)
90-day mortality	105/199 (52.8)	103/199 (51.8)	0.84	1.0 (−8.8 to 10.8)	0.98 (0.81 to 1.18)
Less severe septic shock					
28-day mortality	65/182 (35.7)	52/196 (26.5)	0.05	9.2 (−0.1 to 18.5)	0.74 (0.55 to 1.01)
90-day mortality	83/180 (46.1)	69/193 (35.8)	0.04	10.4 (0.4 to 20.3)	0.78 (0.61 to 0.99)

* Patients with more severe septic shock were defined as those who required at least 15 µg of norepinephrine per minute or the equivalent at the time of randomization. Those with less severe septic shock were defined as those who required 5 to 14 µg of norepinephrine per minute or the equivalent at the time of randomization.

† Two-sided P values are based on Pearson's chi-square test.

noradrenaline among patients with septic shock who were treated with catecholamine vasopressors. They noted that vasopressin was superior in a subgroup of patients with less severe shock (Table 7).

The Bottom line for choice of vasoactive drug for shock

- Catecholamines seem equivalent for major outcomes
- Safety profile and efficacy of noradrenaline may be best overall and in cardiac patients
- Vasopressin in low fixed dose a safe and effective alternative

Early Goal Directed Therapy (EDGT)

An earlier paper by Rivers[18] suggested that targeting a $ScvO_2$ of > 70% and an HCT of > 30%, over and above the conventional hemodynamics, decreases mortality. This was in the context of patients presenting with septic shock in the emergency department. Later another paper showed some benefit of the targeting lactate in addition to the conventional hemodynamic parameters.[19] In the last two years, three large RCTs have examined this[20–22] and all three failed to show any improvement in outcomes. This has been interpreted in many ways. The most quoted reasoning for this lack of improvement is that emergency medicine departments have become good at early resuscitation and giving early antibiotics, and this lead to a sustained decrease in mortality, regardless of the additional use of protocols or $ScvO_2$ targets.

Bottom line: In septic shock presenting to emergency department, rapid administration of antibiotics and standard resuscitation give similar results to protocolized EGDT.

Other Hemodynamic Studies

Sometimes studies give results which go against conventional thought. It is difficult to change established practices based on these studies, but practitioners should at least be aware of these studies, and decide for themselves the validity of continuing or altering their existing practise patterns.

Fluid Bolus in Sepsis

The first surprising study was the FEAST study[23] that was evaluating the role of albumin versus saline in septic children. Patients were divided into hypotensive and non-hypotensive, and almost as an afterthought, a third arm of "no fluid bolus" was included in the non-hypotensive group. As the trial progressed, the data and safety monitoring committee recommended halting recruitment after 3141 of the projected 3600 non-hypotensive children were enrolled. This was because the non-hypotensive children receiving either crystalloid or colloid fluid bolus were dying in larger numbers than those not receiving fluid bolus. There were multiple analysis of this, but it appeared to be a true effect. The administration of fluid bolus to non-hypotensive septic children increased mortality. It's difficult to know how to project the data of septic African children with tropical illness to the normal septic patients in the adult ICU, but at the minimum, one needs to question the role of giving fluid bolus to these patients before hypotension develops.

In a review, Hilton and Bellomo pointed out that "as of 25 May 2011, no studies existed comparing the initial resuscitation of patients with sepsis or septic shock with fluid boluses versus no fluid boluses".[24] The medical community had always presumed that fluids were needed and never tested whether administration of fluid bolus actually made any clinical difference.

IABP in Cardiogenic Shock

The Intra-aortic balloon pump (IABP) is a time-honored technique used in cardiogenic shock, presumed to work by decreasing afterload and also by increasing diastolic coronary perfusion pressure. Without being subjected to a proper RCT, it became a grade 1 recommendation, though recent observational studies have questioned this strong recommendation. When this was finally studied in an RCT (IABP-Shock II)[25] among patients with cardiogenic shock awaiting revascularization, the investigators could find no mortality benefit by using IABP (Figure 15). Other than a benefit among patients less than 50 years old, they could find no subgroup benefit in any other parameter or outcome. One waits to see what the impact of this trial will be on clinical practice. Either further trials will delineate which group of cardiogenic shock patients benefit from IABP, or such as the pulmonary artery catheter, it will slowly disappear from practice.

The above RCT looked at 600 patients in cardiogenic shock after AMI who went on to receive either PCI or CABG. A recent meta-analysis[26] of 625 patients from 8 RCTs evaluated the role of pre-operative IABP in patients undergoing CABG. Though none of the individual trials showed a benefit, the meta-analysis showed an overall 30 day mortality benefit.

Mechanical Ventilation

Theoretical and Pathophysiological Considerations

In the early years of mechanical ventilation, the primary aim was to correct hypoxemia and hypercarbia. Over time, the focus changed to prevention or reversal of respiratory muscle fatigue and "lung protection". The act of subjecting the lung to positive pressure with fixed flows or pressures is inherently unphysiological. Lung injury can result and this can then lead to prolonging or worsening the illness. This is now seen as a major factor in determining outcomes in ventilated patients. The ARDS lungs have been described as

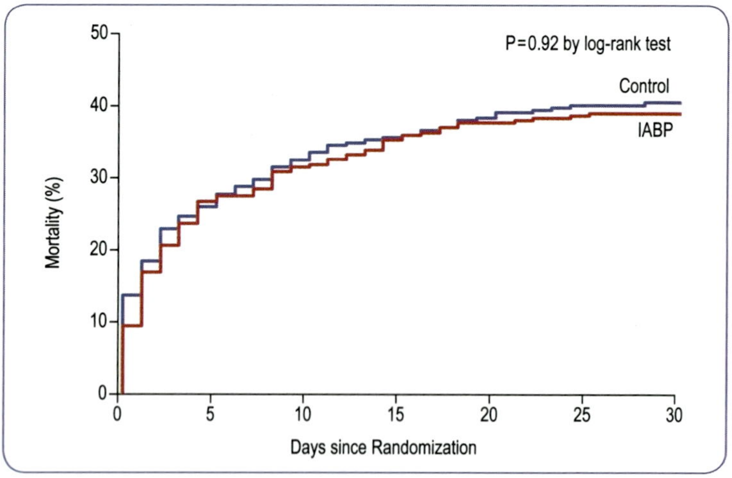

Figure 15. Mortality in IABP-Shock[25]

sponge lungs and baby lungs. This means, like a wet sponge, some of the alveolar airspaces are open, and others are shut. Since much of the lung is involved, the volume of lung which is participating in ventilation and gas exchange is reduced to the size of a baby's lung. Using normal tidal volumes will be injurious in these baby lungs. The underlying concept is to use high expiratory pressures to prevent the alveoli from collapsing and use relatively low inspiratory pressures to prevent over-distension in the ventilated alveoli. The recent studies on mechanical ventilation cover the following questions:

- What is the optimal way of ventilating a patient with ARDS?
- Which weaning technique results in fastest and most successful extubation?
- What is the role of NIV and of early tracheotomy?

Evidence

ARDS

ARDS was first described by Ashbaugh and Petty[27] and its definition and recognition have since evolved. The current Berlin definition[28] is now used for most research.

The ARDS studies are an example of an EBM Success Story. Commenting on research in ARDS, Gattinoni stated[29] "it is important to emphasize how the entire research on this topic may represent one of the best examples of translational research in the field of critical care medicine, with particular regard to the harmful effect of lung hyperinflation and tidal volume setting."

The classic ARDS-Net[30] was a National Institute of Health (NIH) sponsored trial. It involved 861 patients in USA and the trial was stopped prematurely as results were so favourable in the low tidal volume group in the interim analysis. It is worth looking at the trial in some detail. One group got "conventional" ventilation with tidal volume (TV): 12 mL/kg predicted weight and peak airway pressure (PIP) < 50 cm H_2O, while the other group got "protective" ventilation with TV: 6mL/kg predicted weight and PIP < 30 cm H_2O. (This translates to ~5 and 11 mL/Kg actual body weight or approx TV of 350-400 mL vs. 700-800 mL for the average sized patient). There was a lower mortality in the low TV group (31% vs. 39.8%, $P = 0.007$) (Table 8 and Figure 16). The trial raised many concerns about the unphysiological nature of the low TV, the need for increased sedation and the inappropriately high TV and PAP in the control arm. However, this protocol became the standard settings for the control arm of later ARDS trials and in each case was associated with a low mortality of 27.5-31.5%. Given this low mortality in trial after trial, it is worth accepting the ARDS-Net protocol as the default way to ventilate patients with ARDS.

Table 8. Main Outcomes in ARDS-Net Trial[31]			
Variable	**Group Receiving Lower Tidal Volumes**	**Group Receiving Traditional Tidal Volumes**	**P Value**
Death before discharge home and breathing without assistance (%)	31.0	39.8	0.007
Breathing without assistance by day 28 (%)	65.7	55.0	<0.001
No. of ventilator-free days, days 1 to 28	12±11	10±11	0.007
Barotrauma, days 1 to 28 (%)	10	11	0.43
No. of days without failure of nonpulmonary organs or systems, days 1 to 28			

*Plus–minus values are means ±SD. The number of ventilator-free days is the mean number of days from day 1 to day 28 on which the patient had been breathing without assistance for at least 48 consecutive hours. Barotrauma was defined as any new pneumothorax, pneumomediastinum, or subcutaneous emphysema, or a pneumatocele that was more than 2 cm in diameter. Organ and system failures were defined as described in the Methods section.

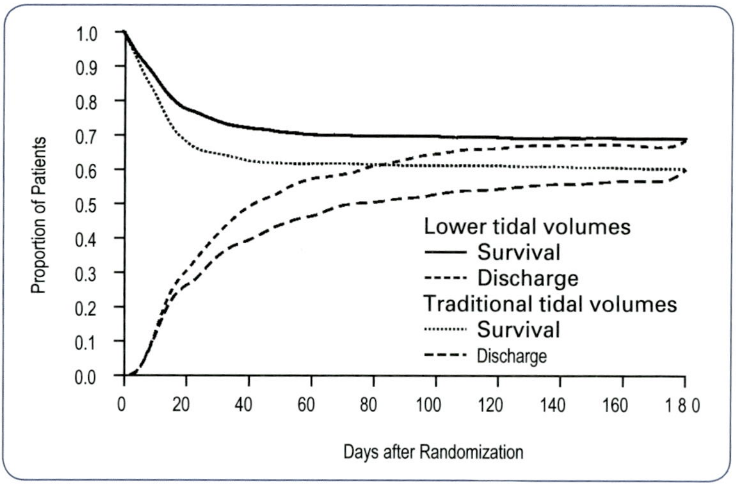

Figure 16. Mortality in ARDS-Net Trial[31]

The ARDS-Net Protocol

Five basic components:

- Volume control ventilation
- Low tidal volume (6 mL/kg ideal body weight)
- Low plateau airway pressure (< 30 cm H_2O)
- Simultaneous escalation of FIO_2 and PEEP to prevent hypoxemia

- Avoidance of hypercarbia and acidosis by increasing respiratory rate and correction of acidosis with HCO_3

PEEP in ARDS

The next issue to resolve in ARDS was whether one should opt for high or low PEEP. Three trials[31–33] looked at this and a meta-analysis of these trials[34] concluded that treatment with higher versus lower levels of PEEP was not associated with improved hospital survival. However, higher levels were associated with improved survival among the subgroup of patients with ARDS (Table 9 and Figure 17).

Fluid / Monitoring Strategy in ARDS

The FACTT trial[35] looked at whether a liberal or a restrictive fluid strategy was associated with improved outcomes and whether the fluid administration should be monitored by a central venous pressure (CVP) catheter or a PAC. They found no significant difference in the primary outcome of 60 day mortality (Figure 18), but they noted the conservative strategy shortened the duration of mechanical ventilation and intensive care without increasing non-pulmonary organ failures. However, a later retrospective analysis of this data showed that patients in the restrictive fluid group had more cognitive dysfunction after recovery Figure 19.[36]

ARDS: Life-Threatening Hypoxemia

Three reviews[37–39] have looked at this in detail and found no evidence to suggest that reversal of hypoxemia improves outcomes. This goes against conventional thinking, but highlights the concept that it is ongoing lung damage and subsequent organ dysfunction rather than hypoxemia which is the main cause of mortality in ARDS. Techniques which have been studied which improve oxygenation but not mortality include recruitment maneuvers (RM) and inhaled nitric oxide (NO). Multiple observational studies suggest RM is most effective when used early and in severe ARDS. Three large multicenter clinical trials found no significant difference in mortality rates, though recent trials reveal significant benefits in multiple secondary outcomes. Several RCTs have evaluated inhaled nitric oxide and found no survival benefit, though they noted improved oxygenation in the first 4 days. A meta-analysis of 12 RCTs raised safety concerns as they showed a trend toward increased mortality rates with inhaled NO and significantly increased risk for renal dysfunction.

ARDS: Glucocorticoids

Steroids are presumed to prevent progress to severe and persistent ALI/ARDS. Large clinical trials have shown no survival benefit. There have been initial improvements in oxygenation

Table 9. Effect of PEEP on Clinical Outcomes in ARDS[35]

	All Patients				With ARDS				Without ARDS			
	No. (%)				No. (%)				No. (%)			
Out comes	Higher PEEP (n = 1136)	Lower PEEP (n = 1163)	Adjusted RR (95% CI)[a]	P Value	Higher PEEP (n = 951)	Lower PEEP (n = 941)	Adjusted RR (95% CI)[a]	P Value	Higher PEEP (n = 184)	Lower PEEP (n = 220)	Adjusted RR (95% CI)[a]	P Value
Death in hospital	374 (32.9)	409 (35.2)	0.94 (0.86 to 1.04)	.25	324 (34.1)	368 (39.1)	0.90 (0.81 to 1.00)	.049	50 (27.2)	44 (19.4)	1.37 (0.98 to 1.92)	.07
Death in ICU[b]	324 (28.5)	381 (32.8)	0.87 (0.78 to 0.97)	.01	288 (30.3)	344 (36.6)	0.85 (0.76 to 0.95)	.001	36 (19.6)	37 (16.8)	1.07 (0.74 to 1.55)	.71
Pneumothorax between day 1 and day 28[c]	87 (7.7)	75 (6.5)	1.19 (0.89 to 1.60)	.24	80 (8.4)	64 (6.8)	1.25 (0.94 to 1.68)	.13	7 (3.8)	11 (5.0)	0.72 (0.37 to 1.39)	.33
Death after pneumothoraxe[c]	43 (3.8)	40 (3.5)	1.11 (0.73 to 1.69)	.63	41 (4.3)	35 (3.7)	1.20 (0.79 to 1.81)	.39	2 (1.1)	5 (2.3)	0.44 (0.08 to 2.35)[e]	.34
Days with unassisted breathing between day 1 and day 28, median (10R)[d]	13 (0 to 22)	11 (0 to 21)	0.64 (-0.12 to 1.39)[e]	.10	12 (0-21)	7 (0-20)	1.22 (0.39 to 2.05)[e]	.004	17 (0-23)	19 (5.5-24)	-1.74 (-3.60 to 0.11)[e]	.07
Total use of rescue therapies	138 (12.2)	216 (18.6)	0.64 (0.54 to 0.75)	<.001	130 (13.7)	200 (21.3)	0.63 (0.53 to 0.75)	<.001	8 (4.4)	16(7.3)	0.60 (0.25 to 1.43)[g]	.25
Death after rescue therapy[f]	85 (7.5)	132 (11.3)	0.65 (0.52 to 0.80)	<.001	82 (8.6)	124 (13.2)	0.66 (0.52 to 0.82)	<.001	3 (1.6)	8 (3.6)	0.37 (0.10 to 1.46)[g]	.15
Use of vasopressors	722 (63.6)	759 (65.3)	0.93 (0.75 to 1.14)[g]	.49	627 (65.9)	647 (68.8)	0.90 (0.72 to 1.13)[g]	.37	95 (51.6)	111 (50.5)	0.92 (0.56 to 1.50)[g]	.72

Abbreviations: ARDS, acute respiratory distress syndrome; CI, confidence interval; ICU, intensive care unit; IQR, interquartile range, PEEP, positive end-expiratory pressure; RR, relative risk

[a] Multivariable regression with the outcome of Interest as dependent variable; PEEP group, age, probability of dying in hospital derived from prognostic scores at baseline, severe sepsis at baseline, and trial as independent variables; and hospital as a random effect.

[b]Patients who died before being discharged from the Intensive care unit for the first time up to day 60.

[c]Defined as the need for chest tube drainage.

[d]Median number of days of unassisted breathing to day 28 after randomization, assuming a patient arrives and remains free of assisted breathing for at least 2 consecutive calendar days after initiation of unassisted breathing.

[e]Coefficient from a corresponding linear regression model using the same independent variables and random effect as the above-described log-binomial model; for example, a coeffident of 122 means that patients in the group treated with higher PEEP have, on average. 122 days more of unassisted breathing daring the first 28 days compared with patients in the group treated with lower PFFP.

[f]As defined in each trial; rescue therapies included in the Assessment of Low Tidal Volume and Elevated End-Expiratory Pressure to Obviate Lung Injury and the Lung Open Ven¬tilation to Decrease Mortality in the Acute Respiratory Distress Syndrome studies: inhaled nitric oxide, prone ventilation, high-frequency oscillation, high-frequency jet ventilation. extracorporeal membrane oxygenation, partial liquid ventilation, and surfactant therapy. Rescue therapies Included in the Expiratory Pressure Study: prone ventilation. inhaled nitric oxide, and almitrine bismesylate.

[g]Adjusted odds ratio substitutes for relative risk, because the corresponding log-binomial model did not converge.

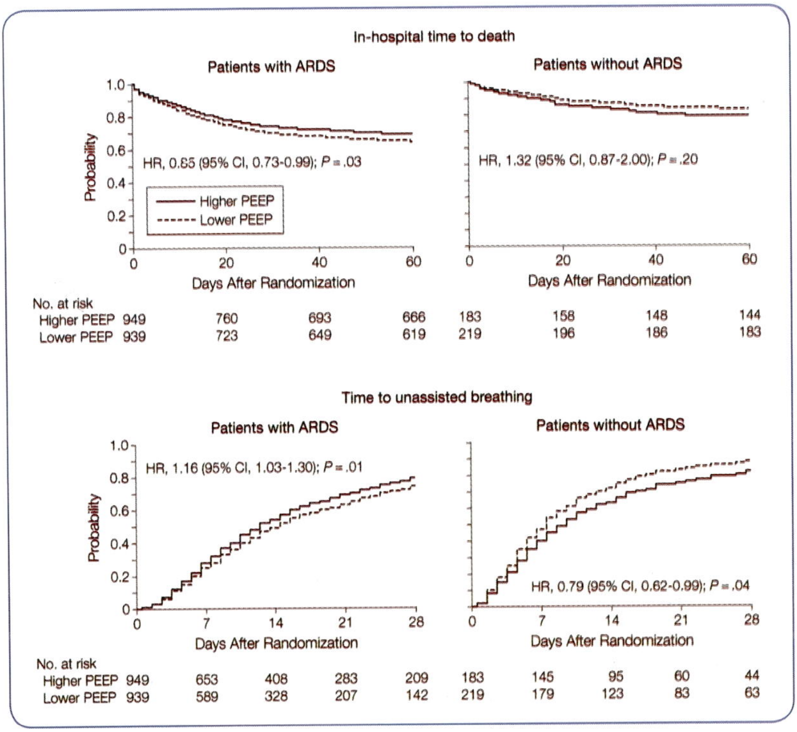

Figure 17. Effect of PEEP on Clinical Outcomes in ARDS[35]

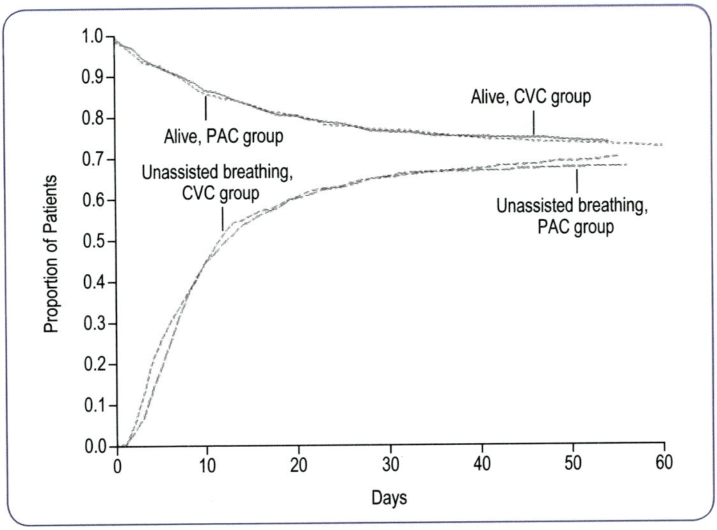

Figure 18. FACTT Trial. Outcome data[36]

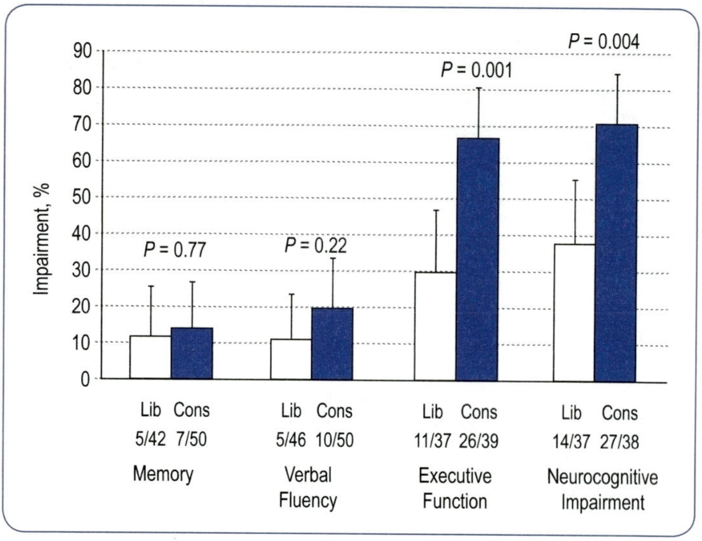

Figure 19. FACTT Trial. Cognitive outcomes[37]

and lung injury scores, but also delayed deterioration due to increased incidence of serious neuromyopathic events. Surprisingly, the larger trials did not show increased risk for infections.

ARDS and Prone Position Ventilation

Initially there was no demonstrated survival benefit in hundreds of patients enrolled in four randomized clinical trials. However, the recent PROSEVA trial,[40] showed a clear survival benefit among patients with severe ARDS (Figure 20). In this trial patients assigned to the prone group had to be turned to the prone position within the 1st hour after randomization. They were placed in a completely prone position for at least 16 consecutive hours. Standard ICU beds were used for all patients.

ARDS: High Frequency Oscillation Ventilation (HFOV) and Extra Corporeal Membrane Oxygenation (ECMO)

The underlying principle behind these techniques is to minimize damage to the lung or to rest the lung. If high PEEP and low TV is protective to the lung, why not pick just one pressure that recruits all the alveoli but does not over-distend them. This allows gas exchange to occur by diffusion with an oscillator facilitating diffusion of gas in the airway, rather than using tidal ventilation to move gas to the alveoli. Similarly, ECMO aims at allowing gas exchange

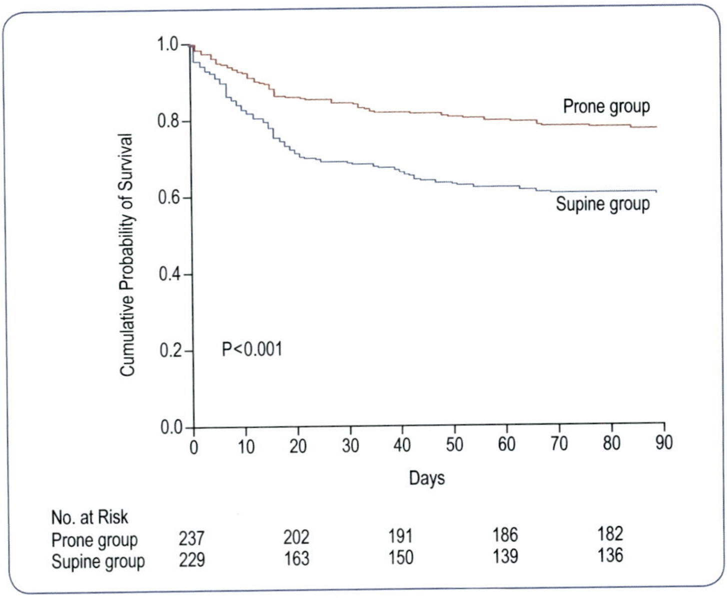

Figure 20. PROSEVA Trial. Outcome data[41]

extra-corporally, thus, minimizing the need for alveolar ventilation and limiting subsequent lung injury.

After some small trials, two large trials evaluated HFOV, the OSCILLATE[41] and the OSCAR trial.[42] Disappointingly, the former actually was associated with a higher mortality and the latter showed no advantage over conventional ventilation.

Only one RCT[43] has examined the demanding technique of ECMO. This study is slightly difficult to interpret. Overall the patients in the ECMO arm did better, but many in this arm did better despite not receiving ECMO. The most appropriate interpretation of this study is that centers which have the volume and the expertise to look after ARDS patients and use ECMO, have better outcomes than centers that have a lower volume of ARDS patients.

ARDS: Bottom Line

- Use low TV and PAP as a default setting.
- In severe ARDS, high PEEP may be advantageous.
- Prone position ventilation is beneficial in severe ARDS.
- Techniques for reversing critical hypoxemia such as NO or RM should only be used as rescue techniques and not as routine part of management.

- Alternatives such as HFOV and ECMO need further evaluation to identify how best to use them. Currently, their use should be limited to centers with enough experience and expertise, or in the context of patients being part of an RCT further evaluating these techniques.
- The below Figure 21 suggests how to align the therapeutic technique to the severity of the illness.

Weaning

Weaning is the process of moving from full control ventilation to spontaneous unassisted breathing and extubation. For short-term ventilation, this is rarely a problem and the patients can rapidly be weaned from the ventilator and extubated. For patients whose recovery is slow, various weaning modes and strategies have been studied. Successful weaning is, when the process is rapid and there is no failure requiring reintubation and ventilation. The following are the main studies in this area.

The first two classic weaning trials were by Brochard and by Estaban. Brochards' trial,[44] looked at 109 patients (T piece (TP)=35, SIMV=43 and PSV=31) and noted less failures with PSV than with the other two modes.

Estaban's trial,[45] was larger (*n* =546). They looked at 4 strategies (SIMV vs. PSV vs. intermittent TP vs. once daily TP) and noted that the T –piece option had more success.

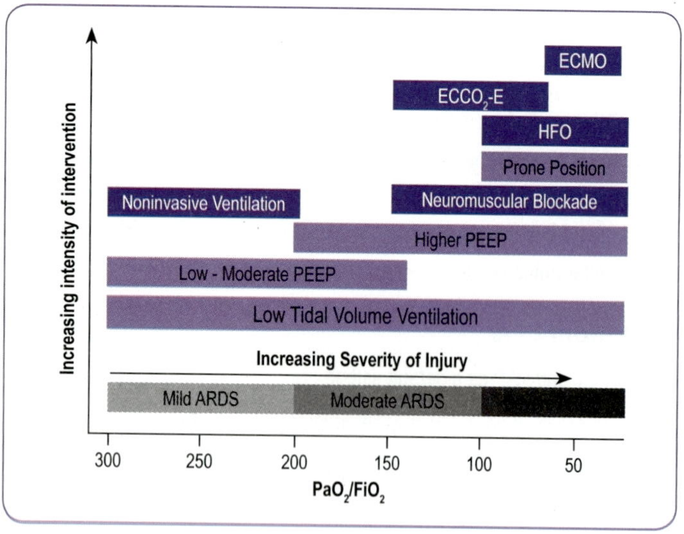

Figure 21. Suggestion how to align the therapeutic technique to the severity of the illness

Since then, there have been a series of trials comparing various modes. The principle findings are summarized.

- Perren: ICM 2002;1058-63: PSV 30 vs. 120 min: equal success.
- Estaban AJRCCM 1997;156:162-66: 2 hr trial T-Piece vs. PSV : More failure with TP.
- Koh J Crit Care 2000;15:41-45: PSV vs. PSV + T-piece: equal success.
- Matic Croation Med J 2004;45:162-66: Repeated daily 2 hr T-Piece vs. PSV: PSV more successful.
- Vitacca ARJCCM 2001;164:225-30: COPD: T-Piece vs. PSV: Equal success.

Another classic trial by Kollef,[46] evaluated the role of protocol-directed (n = 179) vs. physician directed (n = 178) weaning from mechanical ventilation. They showed that protocol-guided weaning of mechanical ventilation, as performed by nurses and respiratory therapists, was safe and led to extubation more rapidly than physician-directed weaning. Since then, there have been a series of similar trials and a Cochrane systematic review and meta-analysis[47] concluded that there is evidence of a reduction in the duration of mechanical ventilation, weaning, and stay in the intensive care unit when standardised weaning protocols are used, but there is significant heterogeneity amongst the studies (Figure 22 below).

Bottom Line: Weaning by PSV or T-piece is preferable to SIMV and the use of protocols speeds up the weaning process.

Non Invasive Ventilation

This is a technique of ventilating a patient with a mask. It has many potential advantages, mainly avoiding intubation and sedation. However, it is not as efficient and failure will require tracheal intubation. Delay in shifting from NIV to intubation can result in significant patient deterioration and even a cardio respiratory arrest. It is therefore, important to be judicious when using NIV. Below are the main studies that examine the role in various forms of respiratory failure.

The following is a summary of the trials evaluating NIV. The first classic trial was again by Brochard[48] looking at the role of NIV in 85 patients with acute exacerbation of COPD. The patients in the NIV arm of the study needed less intubation (26 vs. 74%: $P < 0.001$), had less complications (16 vs. 48 %: $P = 0.001$), a shorter hospital stay (23 vs. 35 days, $P = 0.005$) and a lower in-hospital mortality (9 vs. 29%: $P = 0.02$). A subsequent meta-analysis[49] confirmed both the lower risk of a composite endpoint of mortality, intubation and intolerance to treatment (Figure 23).

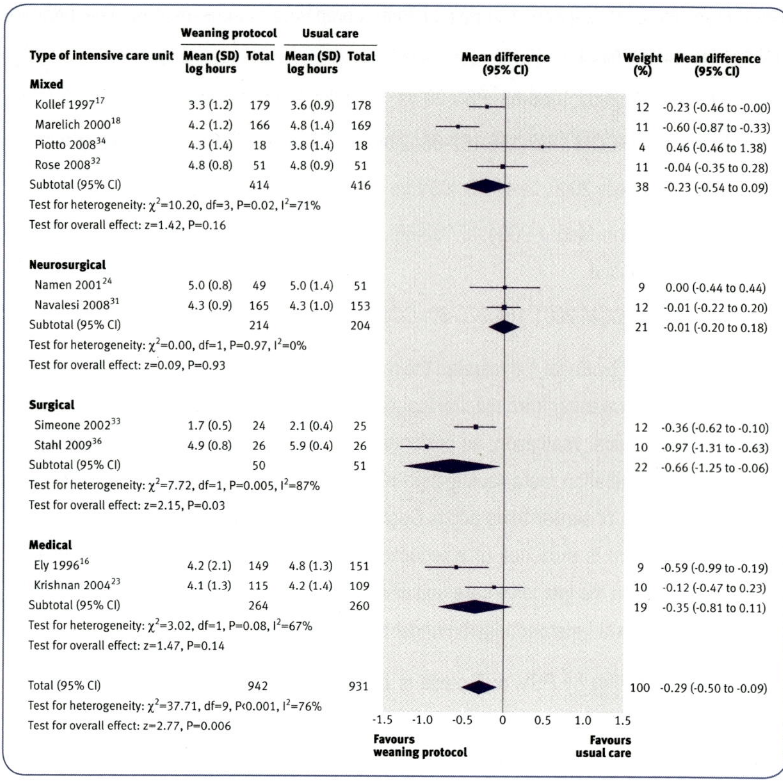

Figure 22. Meta-analysis of weaning by protocol trials

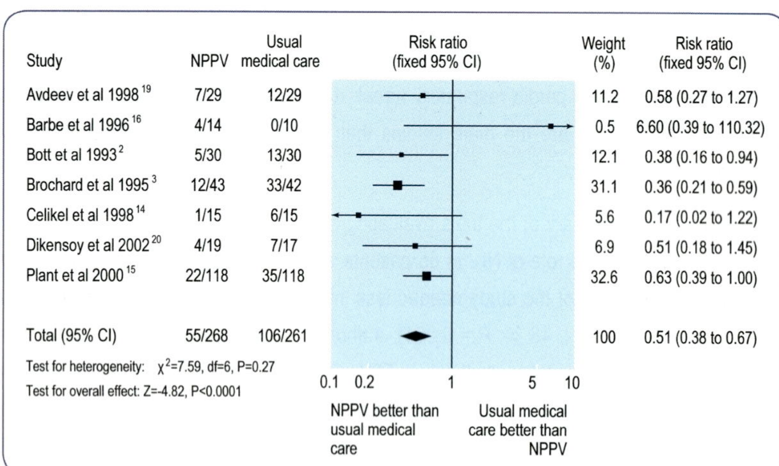

Figure 23. Meta-analysis of NIV in COPD[49]

Hilbert evaluated the role of NIV in 52 immune compromised[50] patients with chest infiltrates and hypoxemia, and concluded that in selected immunosuppressed patients with pneumonitis and acute respiratory failure, early initiation of noninvasive ventilation is associated with significant reductions in the rates of endotracheal intubation and serious complications and an improved likelihood of survival to hospital discharge.

The evidence for benefit of NIV in Cardiogenic Pulmonary Edema is less uniform. An earlier meta-analysis[51] showed that CPAP reduces mortality and there is a trend towards reduced mortality after bi-level NIPPV and also showed that CPAP and BiPAP reduce intubation.

A later large RCT[52] in 1069 patients compared O_2 vs. CPAP vs. NIV and found no significant difference in 7 day mortality or intubation rates. They did note less dyspnea, lower heart rate, acidosis and CO_2 at 1 hour and concluded that among patients with acute cardiogenic pulmonary edema, noninvasive ventilation induces a more rapid improvement in respiratory distress and metabolic disturbance than does standard oxygen therapy but has no effect on short-term mortality.

A meta-analysis for NIV for Weaning[53] found decreased mortality, pneumonia, and shorter length of stay (LOS) in ICU and hospital.

NIV: Bottom line

- There is strong evidence of efficacy in acute exacerbation of COPD, acute cardiogenic pulmonary edema, immune compromised and in facilitation from weaning in COPD.
- There is intermediate evidence of efficacy in asthma, COPD with CAP, hypoxemic respiratory failure, post operative respiratory failure and when used for palliation in patients with Do Not Intubate and/or Do Not Resuscitate orders (DNI-DNR).

Tracheostomy

The literature on the timing of tracheostomy is disappointing. There is a widespread perception that early tracheostomy is beneficial in those estimated to require prolonged ventilation. The first small RCT[54] was encouraging with the early (48 hours) tracheostomy group having a lower mortality (31.7% vs. 61.7%), pneumonia (5% vs. 25%) and accidental extubations (0 vs. 6) compared to the late (day 14-16) tracheostomy group. The early group showed significantly shorter LOS of both mechanical ventilation and ICU stay.

The larger TracMan Trial[55] showed that early tracheostomy reduces sedative use but did not affect mortality. It also showed that there were a significant number of unnecessary tracheostomies in the early group (Table 10).

Table 10. Primary and Secondary Outcomes in TracMan Trial[55]

	No. (%) of Patients [95% CI]			Absolute Risk Reduction for Early vs Late (95% CI), %	Relative Risk for Early vs Late (95% CI)	P Value for Fisher Exact Test
	Early (n = 451)	Late (n = 448)	Total (n = 899)			
Status at 30 d (primary outcome) Died	139 (30.8) [26.7 to 35.2]	141 (31.5) [27.3 to 35.9]	280 (31.2) [28.2 to 34.3]	0.7 (5.4 to 6.7)	0.98 (0.81 to 1.19)	89
Status at ICU discharge[a]						
No. of patients	448	445	893			
Died	133 (29.7) [25.6 to 34.1]	132 (29.7) [25.6 to 34.1]	265 (29.7) [26.8 to 32.8]	0.0 (6.0 to 6.0)	1.00 (0.82 to 1.22)	>.99
Status at hospital discharge[b]						
No. of patients	424	436	860			
Died	168 (39.6) [35.1 to 44.4]	180 (41.3) [36.8 to 46.0]	348 (40.5) [37.2 to 43.8]	1.7 (4.9 to 8.2)	0.96 (0.82 to 1.13)	.63
Status at 1 y[c]						
No. of patients	451	443	894			
Died	207 (45.9) [41.4 to 50.5]	217 (49.0) [44.4 to 53.6]	424 (47.4) [44.2 to 50.7]	3.1 (3.5 to 9.6)	0.94 (0.82 to 1.08)	.38
Status at 2 y[d]						
No. of patients	451	443	894			
Died	230 (51.0) [46.4 to 55.6]	238 (53.7) [49.1 to 58.3]	468 (52.3) [49.1 to 55.6]	0.7 (3.8 to 9.3)	0.95 (0.84 to 1.08)	.42

Abbreviation: ICU, intensive care unit.

[a]Status at critical care unit discharge not available for 6 patients (3 early, 3 late).

[b]Status at hospital discharge not available for 39 patients (27 early, 12 late).

[c]Status at 1 y not available for 5 patients (5 late).

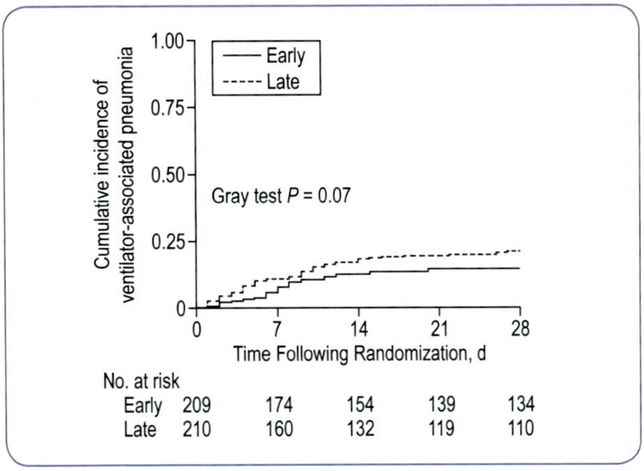

Figure 24. Pneumonia rate in early vs late tracheostomy[56]

The Terragni trial[56] in 600 patients showed similar VAP rates (Figure 24) but more ventilator and ICU free days in the early group. However, they also noted a high incidence of adverse events related to the tracheostomy (39% both groups) and they suggest that a tracheotomy should not be performed earlier than after 13 to 15 days of endotracheal intubation.

There have been further meta-analysis of these trials[57] failing to show a benefit of early tracheostomy. One meta-analysis did show an improvement,[58] but that was later retracted[59] due to methodological problems. This has been republished in Feb 2015,[60] but failed to show a mortality benefit in the early tracheostomy group.

Bottom Line: Routine early tracheostomy in those estimated to require prolonged ventilation is not justified based on the present evidence.

Renal Replacement Therapy

Theoretical and Pathophysiological Considerations

There are two types of acute renal failure (ARF) in an ICU patient. That which presents to an intensivist and that which presents to a nephrologist. The approach to each is different.

The first type is much more common. A patient has a major illness and despite resuscitation, progresses to oligoanuria and azotemia. From a global pathophysiological perspective, ARF as part of Multi Organ Failure (MOF) is not really a disease of the kidney. Rather, it is a renal manifestation of a systemic illness, and dialysis is not going to reverse the problem. Once renal failure occurs, over a period of time, classic ARF complications such as pulmonary edema or acidosis and hyperkalemia may occur. These may then worsen the physiology and subsequently worsen the MOF. Diuretic use will maintain urine production and limit the fluid volume overload. Simply instituting renal replacement therapy (RRT) in this setting is rarely curative. It is here that the role, choice, timing and dose of renal replacement therapy are unclear. The studies discussed in this chapter look at the role of diuretics and the options for renal replacement therapy in these patients with ARF as a part of shock and MOF. The options are Intermittent RRT (hemodialysis) or continuous RRT (hemofiltration) and standard versus high intensity RRT.

The other type of ARF is a less common one. A patient has developed renal failure and presents to a nephrologist prior to ICU admission. The patient then develops complications such as pulmonary edema or hyperkalemia and acidosis. This needs standard ICU management of the above. If indicated, dialysis will correct the complications. The dialysis needs to be continued regularly till such time as the kidney has recovered. Patients with Chronic Renal failure (CRF) too may occasionally present similarly, and the decompensation is often triggered by an infection, an episode of cardiac failure, or due to delayed or missed dialysis. They generally recover quickly with appropriate treatment and dialysis.

Some other considerations need to be kept in mind. Patients with established renal failure can have further worsening of renal function or delayed renal recovery, if all pre renal factors are not constantly corrected. Similarly, nephrotoxic factors such as hemoglobinuria, myoglobinuria or hyperuricemia need to be rapidly corrected. Nephrotoxic drugs should not be used even if "the kidney has anyway gone" as they will increase the risk of long term loss of renal function.

Physiologically, there is little plausibility of introducing certain standard renal treatments in the ICU patients with ARF. There is little reason or evidence to routinely use iron and erythropoietin, calcium and vitamin D or bicarbonate among patients with acute renal failure.

Evidence

Renal dose dopamine

A low, non inotropic-vasoconstrictor dose of dopamine was shown to improve renal flow and function in small physiological studies, and this lead to its widespread use among patients with renal risk or dysfunction. It was tested in a classic ANZICS trial[61] and found to have no impact on any clinically meaningful outcome such as mortality, renal failure or need for renal replacement therapy. It has since disappeared from routine practice.

Diuretics

The role of high-dose loop diuretics in the prevention and management of oliguric or anuric ARF is uncertain. A meta-analysis[62] concluded that loop diuretics were not associated with improved survival benefit in acute renal failure, despite reduction in oliguric period and high probability of a significant reduction in dialysis numbers. It would appear that diuretics should be used in appropriate doses to maintain a non oliguric state and to prevent volume overload. The routine use of higher doses for prevention of complications is unclear.

HD versus CRRT

Four studies have shown no overall superiority.[63–66] In the BEST trial, the choice of continuous renal replacement therapy (CRRT) was not an independent predictor of hospital survival or dialysis-free hospital survival. However, the choice of CRRT was a predictor of dialysis independence at hospital discharge among survivors (OR: 3.333, 95% CI:1.845 - 6.024, $P<0.0001$). Currently, the choice should be based on patients need and hemodynamic stability.

High versus Standard dose or intensity of RRT

An earlier trial by Ronco[67] suggested that high-dose continuous veno-venous hemofiltration (CVVH) is associated with better outcomes. After that two large trials[68,69] have tested the effect of standard vs. high intensity RRT and failed to show a convincing mortality or other clinical benefit.

Early versus late

Classic indications for dialysis are hyperkalemia, acidosis and respiratory failure from pulmonary edema. Rarely a patient with CRF presents very late with encephalopathy, pericarditis and GI bleed, and these too require dialysis. One could consider dialysis "early" if it is initiated before any of these classic indications occur. That is, it is started purely on the basis of an increasing azotemia or a low urine output. Part of the difficultly arises in predicting the timing and severity of AKI. It does not make sense to dialyze someone with a renal injury which is going to have an uncomplicated recovery, as RRT carries risk of complications, besides being expensive, time consuming and resource intense. On the other hand, it is preferable to prevent complications rather than treat them.

At present good evidence around the best time to initiate RRT in AKI is still lacking. The first study looking at early intervention was in 2003 and the study showed promise. In this study of 44 cardiac surgery patients with a creatinine of > 2.5 mg, the 21 who received prophylactic peri-operative dialysis had much lower morbidity and risk of mortality (4.8 vs. 30.4) than the 23 patients who did not.[70] Though encouraging, the small numbers and the high mortality make one a little cautious about fully accepting the results. Another trial looked at timing of RRT in cardiac surgery patients[71] concluded that timing of the start of treatment for acute renal failure following cardiac surgery should be determined by the decrease in urine volume (<30 mL / hour vs. < 20 mL/hour) and not the levels of serum creatinine. Early start of dialysis therapy may help improve the survival of patients with acute renal failure following cardiac surgery. They noted a mortality of 2/14 in the early RRT group versus 12/14 in the late RRT group.

Two studies have compared different strategies in ARF. In both the control group got conventional management with HD while the treatment group got earlier and more intense RRT with CVVH. Ronco studied 80 patients with septic shock.[72] Forty patients got conventional supportive therapy and 40 patients got early isovolemic hemofiltration (EIHF) at 45 mL/kg/h of plasma-water exchange over 6 h followed by CVVH. The authors concluded that among patients with septic shock, EIHF was associated with improved gas exchange, hemodynamics, greater likelihood of successful weaning and greater 28 day survival compared with conventional therapy. Again one is cautious when looking at mortality in a study with a small number of patients. Another similar two centre study failed to show a 28 day reduction in either mortality or on recovery of renal function.[73]

A meta-analysis[74] demonstrated that earlier institution of RRT in critically ill patients with AKI may have a beneficial impact on survival (Figure 25). However, this conclusion is based on heterogeneous studies of variable quality and only two randomised trials. In the absence of new evidence from suitably-designed randomised trials, a definitive treatment recommendation cannot be made.

The Canadian Critical Care trials Group is doing a study on Standard vs. Accelerated Initiation of Renal Replacement Therapy in Acute Kidney Injury (STARRT-AKI) and the results of that will hopefully resolve the question as to whether early RRT improves clinical outcomes.

Two larger studies have shown that outcomes are worse with fluid accumulation, but do not clarify if early RRT to prevent this actually improves outcomes.[75,76]

Bottom Line

- ARF as part of MOF is not a simple form of kidney failure. It is the renal manifestation of a systemic disease and RRT alone will not cure the patient.
- Renal dose dopamine is ineffective and should not be used.

Meta analysis: All 15 studies

Study name	Subroup within study	Statistics for each study				
		Odds ratio	Lower limit	Upper limit	Z-value	P-value
Bouman 2002	Mixed	1.375	0.487	3.884	0.601	0.548
Sugahara 2004	Surgery	0.028	0.003	0.231	-3.318	0.001
Liu 2006	Mixed	0.773	0.460	1.298	-0.974	0.330
Sabater 2008	Mixed	0.055	0.006	0.524	-2.520	0.012
Bagshaw 2010*	Mixed	1.563	0.933	2.619	1.697	0.090
Gettings 1999	Surgery	0.399	0.164	0.973	-2.019	0.043
Elahi 2004	Surgery	0.800	0.273	2.341	-0.407	0.684
Demirkilic 2004	Surgery	0.533	0.183	1.552	-1.154	0.249
Andrade 2007	Mixed	0.100	0.019	0.515	-2.752	0.006
Manche 2008	Surgery	0.051	0.010	0.256	-3.623	0.000
Iyem 2009	Surgery	0.778	0.229	2.644	-0.403	0.687
Shiao 2008	Surgery	0.260	0.110	0.614	-3.075	0.002
Bagshaw 2009 adj	Mixed	1.250	0.915	1.708	1.401	0.161
Wu 2007 adj	Surgical	0.259	0.068	0.988	-1.977	0.048
Carl 2010 adj	Mixed	0.380	0.177	0.816	-2.482	0.013
		0.446	0.276	0.723	--3.279	0.001

Odds ratio and 95% CI

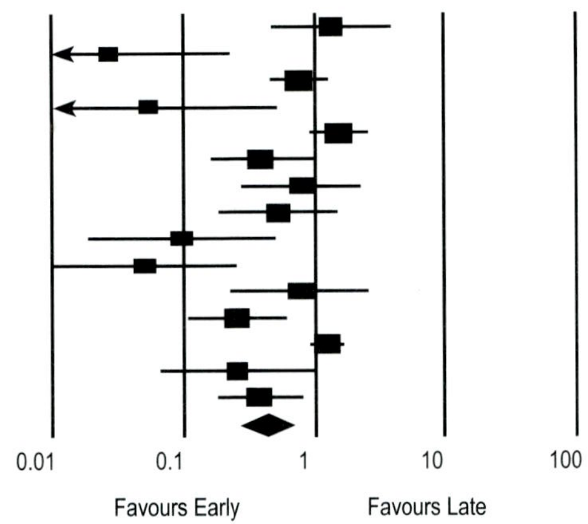

Meta analysis

Figure 25. Effect of Early RRT on outcome[74]

- Diuretics should be used to limit oliguria and fluid overload.
- HD and CRRT appear to have similar clinical outcomes.
- Standard intensity and high intensity RRT appear to have similar outcomes.
- The timing of initiation of RRT is unclear.

Conclusions

This chapter covers most of the important trials for the standard ICU techniques used to keep a patient alive. These trials have also had the most impact in the delivery of critical care in the last decade. The summary boxes at the end of each section represent our interpretation of the data.

References

1. Steven M. Hollenberg Vasoactive drugs in circulatory shock. *Am J Respir Crit Care Med* 2011;183(7):847–55.
2. Asfar P, Meziani F, Hamel JF, *et al.* for the SEPSISPAM Investigators. High versus Low Blood-Pressure Target in Patients with Septic Shock. *N Engl J Med* 2014;370:1583–93.
3. Walsh M, Devereaux PJ, Garg AX, *et al.* Relationship between intraoperative mean arterial pressure and clinical outcomes after non-cardiac surgery. *Anesthesiology* 2013;119:507–15.
4. Dutton RP, Mackenzie CF, Scalea TM. Hypotensive resuscitation during active hemorrhage: impact on in-hospital mortality. *J Trauma* 2002;52(6):1141–46.
5. Morrison CA, Carrick MM, Norman MA, *et al.* Hypotensive resuscitation strategy reduces transfusion requirements and severe postoperativecoagulopathy in trauma patients with hemorrhagic shock: preliminary results of a randomized controlled trial. *J Trauma* 2011;70:652–63.
6. Finfer S, Bellomo R, Boyce N, *et al.* A comparison of albumin and saline for fluid resuscitation in the intensive care unit. *N Engl J Med* 2004;350:2247–56.
7. Guidet B, Martinet O, Boulain T, *et al.* Assessment of hemodynamic efficacy and safety of 6% hydroxyethylstarch 130/0.4 versus 0.9% NaCl fluid replacement in patients with severe sepsis: the CRYSTMAS study. *Crit Care* 2012;16:R94.
8. Hydroxyethyl starch 130/0.4 versus Ringer's acetate in severe sepsis. (Scandinavian Starch for Severe Sepsis/Septic Shock (6S) trial). *N Engl J Med* 2012.DOI: 10.1056/NEJMoa1204242.
9. Myburgh JA, Finfer S, Bellomo R, *et al.* Hydroxyethyl starch or saline for fluid resuscitation in Intensive Care. *N Engl J Med* 2012;367:1901–11.
10. Annane D, Siami S, Jaber S, *et al.* Effects of fluid resuscitation with colloids versus crystalloids on mortality in critically ill patients presenting with hypovolemic shock: the CRISTAL randomized trial. *JAMA* 2013;310:1809–17.
11. Caironi P, Tognoni G, Masson S, *et al.* for the ALBIOS Study Investigators. Albumin replacement in patients with severe sepsis or septic shock. *N Engl J Med* 2014;370:1412–21.
12. Wiedermann and Joannidis. Albumin replacement in severe sepsis or septic shock. *N Engl J Med* 2014;371:83.
13. Annane D, Vignon P, Renault A, *et al.* Norepinephrine plus dobutamine versus epinephrine alone for management of septic shock: a randomised trial. *Lancet* 2007;370:676–84.
14. Myburgh JA, Higgins A, Jovanovska A, *et al.* A comparison of epinephrine and norepinephrine in critically ill patients. *Intensive care medicine* 2008;34:2226–34.

15. De Backer D, Biston P, Devriendt J, *et al.* Comparison of dopamine and norepinephrine in the treatment of shock. *N Engl J Med* 2010;362:779–89.
16. De Backer D, Aldecoa C, Njimi H, *et al.* Dopamine versus norepinephrine in the treatment of septic shock: a meta-analysis. *Crit Care Med* 2012;40:725–30.
17. Russell JA, Walley KR, Singer J, *et al.* Vasopressin versus norepinephrine infusion in patients with septic shock. *N Engl J Med* 2008;358:877–87.
18. Rivers E, Nguyen B, Havstad S, *et al.* Early goal-directed therapy in the treatment of severe sepsis and septic shock. *N Engl J Med* 2001;345:1368–77.
19. Jansen TC, van Bommel J, Schoonderbeek FJ, *et al.* LACTATE study group. Early lactate-guided therapy in intensive care unit patients: a multicenter, open-label, randomized controlled trial. *Am J Respir Crit Care Med* 2010;182(6):752–61.
20. Peake SL, Delaney A, Bailey M, *et al.* Goal-directed resuscitation for patients with early septic shock. *N Engl J Med* 2014;371:1496–1506.
21. The ProCESS Investigators, Yealy DM, Kellum JA, *et al.* A randomized trial of protocol-based care for early septic shock. *N Engl J Med* 2014;370:1683–93.
22. Mouncey PR, Osborn TM, Power GS, *et al.* for the ProMISe Trial Investigators. Trial of early, goal-directed resuscitation for septic shock. *N Engl J Med* 2015;372:1301–11.
23. Maitland K, Kiguli S, Opoka RO, *et al.* for the FEAST Trial Group. Mortality after fluid bolus in African children with severe infection. *N Engl J Med* 2011;364:2483–95.
24. Hilton AK, Bellomo R.. A critique of fluid bolus resuscitation in severe sepsis. *Critical Care* 2012;16:302.
25. Thiele H, Zeymer U, Neumann FJ, *et al.* for the IABP-SHOCK II Trial Investigators. Intraaortic balloon support for myocardial infarction with cardiogenic shock. *N Engl J Med* 2012;367:1287–96.
26. Zangrillo A, Pappalardo F, Dossi R, *et al.* Preoperative intra-aortic balloon pump to reduce mortality in coronary artery bypass graft: a meta-analysis of randomized controlled trials. *Critical Care* 2015;19:10.
27. Ashbaugh DG, Bigelow DB, Petty TL *et al.* Acute Respiratory Distress in Adults. *Lancet* 1967;2:319–23.
28. The ARDS Definition Task Force, Ranieri VM, Rubenfeld GD, *et al.* Acute respiratory distress syndrome: the Berlin Definition. *JAMA* 2012;307:2526–33.
29. Caironi P, Langer T, Gattinoni L. Acute lung injury/acute respiratory distress syndrome pathophysiology: what we have learned from computed tomography scanning. *Curr Opin Crit Care* 2008;14(1):64–9.
30. The Acute Respiratory Distress Syndrome Network. Ventilation with lower tidal volumes as compared with traditional tidal volumes for acute lung injury and the acute respiratory distress syndrome. *N Engl J Med* 2000;342:1301–8.
31. Brower RG, Lanken PN, MacIntyre N, *et al.* Higher versus lower positive end-expiratory pressures in patients with the acute respiratory distress syndrome. *N Engl J Med* 2004;351:327–36.
32. Mercat A, Richard JC, Vielle B, *et al.* Positive end-expiratory pressure setting in adults with acute lung injury and acute respiratory distress syndrome: a randomized controlled trial. Expiratory Pressure (Express) Study Group. *JAMA* 2008;299:646–55.
33. Meade MO, Cook DJ, Guyatt GH, *et al.* Lung Open Ventilation Study Investigators. Ventilation strategy using low tidal volumes, recruitment maneuvers, and high positive end-expiratory pressure for acute lung injury and acute respiratory distress syndrome: a randomized controlled trial. *JAMA* 2008;299:637–45.
34. Briel M, Meade M, Mercat A, *et al.* Higher versus lower positive end-expiratory pressure in patients with acute lung injury and acute respiratory distress syndrome: systematic review and meta-analysis. *JAMA* 2010;303:865–73.
35. National Heart, Lung, and Blood Institute Acute Respiratory Distress Syndrome (ARDS) Clinical Trials Network, Wheeler AP, Bernard GR, *et al.* Pulmonary-artery versus central venous catheter to guide treatment of acute lung injury. *N Engl J Med* 2006;354:2213–24.

36. Mikkelsen ME, Christie JD, Lanken PN, *et al.* The adult respiratory distress syndrome cognitive outcomes study long-term neuropsychological function in survivors of acute lung injury. *Am J Respir Crit Care Med* 2012;185:1307–15.

37. Diaz JV, Brower R, Calfee CS, *et al.* Therapeutic strategies for severe acute lung injury. *Crit Care Med* 2010;38:1644 –50.

38. Pipeling MR, Fan E. Therapies for refractory hypoxemia in acute respiratory distress syndrome. *JAMA* 2010;304:2521–27.

39. Patroniti N, Isgrò S, Zanella A. Clinical management of severely hypoxemic patients. *Critical Care* 2011;17:50–56.

40. Guérin C, Reignier J, Richard JC, *et al.* for the PROSEVA Study Group. Prone positioning in severe acute respiratory distress syndrome. *N Engl J Med* 2013;368:2159–68.

41. Ferguson ND, Cook DJ, Guyatt GH, *et al.* for the OSCILLATE Trial Investigators. High-frequency oscillation in early acute respiratory distress syndrome. *N Engl J Med* 2013;368:795–805.

42. Young D, Lamb SE, Shah S, *et al.* for the OSCAR Study Group. High-frequency oscillation for acute respiratory distress syndrome. *N Engl J Med* 2013;368:806–13.

43. Peek GJ, Mugford M, Tiruvoipati R, *et al.* for the CESAR trial collaboration. Efficacy and economic assessment of conventional ventilatory support versus extracorporeal membrane oxygenation for severe adult respiratory failure (CESAR): a multicentre randomised controlled trial. *Lancet* 2009;374:1351–63.

44. Brochard L, Rauss A, Benito S, *et al.* Comparison of three methods of gradual withdrawal from ventilatory support during weaning from mechanical ventilation. *Am J Respir Crit Care Med* 1994;150:896–903.

45. Esteban A, Frutos F, Tobin MJ, *et al.* A comparison of four methods of weaning patients from mechanical ventilation. *N Engl J Med* 1995;332:345–50.

46. Kollef MH, Shapiro SD, Silver P, *et al.* A randomized, controlled trial of protocol-directed versus physician-directed weaning from mechanical ventilation. *Crit Care Med* 1997; 25:567–74.

47. Blackwood B, Alderdice F, Burns K, *et al.* Use of weaning protocols for reducing duration of mechanical ventilation in critically ill adult patients: Cochrane systematic review and meta-analysis. *BMJ* 2011;342:c7237.

48. Brochard L, Mancebo J, Wysocki M, *et al.* Non-invasive ventilation for acute exacerbations of chronic obstructive pulmonary disease. *N Engl J Med* 1995;333:817–22.

49. Lightowler JV, Wedzicha JA, Elliott MW, *et al.* Non-invasive positive pressure ventilation to treat respiratory failure resulting from exacerbations of chronic obstructive pulmonary disease: Cochrane systematic review and meta-analysis. *BMJ* 2003;326:185.

50. Hilbert G, Gruson D, Vargas F, *et al.* Non-invasive ventilation in immunosuppressed patients with pulmonary infiltrates, fever, and acute respiratory failure. *N Engl J Med* 2001;344:481–87.

51. Peter JV, Moran JL, Phillips-Hughes J, *et al.* Effect of non-invasive positive pressure ventilation (NIPPV) on mortality in patients with acute cardiogenic pulmonary edema: a meta-analysis. *Lancet* 2006;367:1155–63.

52. Gray A, Goodacre S, Newby DE, *et al.* Non-invasive ventilation in acute cardiogenic pulmonary edema. *N Engl J Med* 2008;359:142–151.

53. Burns. The Cochrane Library 2005, Issue 3.

54. Rumbak MJ, Newton M, Truncale T, *et al.* A prospective, randomized, study comparing early percutaneous dilational tracheotomy to prolonged translaryngeal intubation (delayed tracheotomy) in critically ill medical patients. *Crit Care Med* 2004;32:1689–94.

55. Young D, Harrison DA, Cuthbertson BH, *et al.* Effect of early vs. late tracheostomy placement on survival in patients receiving mechanical ventilation: the TracMan randomized trial. *JAMA* 2013;309:2121–29.

56. Terragni PP, Antonelli M, Fumagalli R, *et al.* Early vs. late tracheotomy for prevention of pneumonia in mechanically ventilated adult ICU patients: a randomized controlled trial. *JAMA* 2010;303(15):1483–89.

57. Huang H, Li Y, Ariani F, *et al.* Timing of tracheostomy in critically ill patients: a meta-analysis. *PLoS ONE* 2014 ;9(3): e92981.

58. Effect of early versus late or no tracheostomy on mortality of critically ill patients receiving mechanical ventilation: a systematic review and meta-analysis. *Lancet Respir Med* 2014. Published Online. June 27, 2014.

59. RETRACTED: Effect of early versus late or no tracheostomy on mortality of critically ill patients receiving mechanical ventilation: a systematic review and meta-analysis. *Lancet Respir Med* October 14, 2014(http://www.ncbi.nlm.nih.gov/pubmed/24981963

60. Siempos II, Ntaidou TK, Filippidis FT, *et al.* Effect of early versus late or no tracheostomy on mortality and pneumonia of critically ill patients receiving mechanical ventilation: a systematic review and meta-analysis. *Lancet* 2015;3:150–58.

61. Bellomo R, Chapman M, Finfer S, *et al.* Low-dose dopamine in patients with early renal dysfunction: a placebo-controlled randomised trial. Australian and New Zealand intensive care society (ANZICS) clinical trials group. *Lancet* 2000;356:2139–43.

62. Sampath S, Moran JL, Graham PL, *et al.* The efficacy of loop diuretics in acute renal failure: assessment using Bayesian evidence synthesis techniques. *Crit Care Med* 2007;35:2516–24.

63. Mehta RL, Mc Donald B, Gabbai FB, *et al.* A randomized clinical trial of continuous versus intermittent dialysis for acute renal failure. *Kidney Intl* 2001;60:1154–63.

64. Uchino S, Kellum JA. Beginning and Ending Supportive Therapy for the Kidney (BEST Kidney) Investigators. Acute renal failure in critically ill patients: a multinational, multicenter study. *JAMA* 2005;294: 813–8.

65. Vinsonneau C, Camus C, Combes A, *et al.* Continuous venovenous hemodiafiltration versus intermittent hemodialysis for acute renal failure in patients with multiple-organ dysfunction syndrome: a multicentre randomised trial. *Lancet* 2006;368:379–85.

66. Lins R, Elseviers M, Van der Niepen P, *et al.*; SHARF Investigators: Intermittent versus continuous renal replacement therapy for acute kidney injury patients admitted to the intensive care unit: Results of a randomized clinical trial. *Nephrol Dial Transplant* 2009;24:512–8.

67. Ronco C, Bellomo R, Homel P, *et al.* Effects of different doses in continuous veno-venous hemofiltration on outcomes of acute renal failure: a prospective randomised trial. Lancet 2000;356(9223):26–30.

68. RENAL Trial Intensity of continuous renal-replacement therapy in critically ill patients. *N Engl J Med* 2009;361(17):1627–38.

69. VA/NIH ATN Trial. Intensity of renal support in critically ill patients with acute kidney injury. *N Engl J Med* 2008;359(1):7–20.

70. Durmaz I, Yagdi T, Calkavur T, *et al.* Prophylactic dialysis in patients with renal dysfunction undergoing on-pump coronary artery bypass surgery. *Ann Thorac Surg* 2003;75(3):859–64.

71. Souichi SUGAHARA, Hiromichi SUZUKI. Early start on continuous hemodialysis therapy improves survival rate in patients with acute renal failure following coronary bypass surgery. *Hemodial Int* 2004;8:320–5.

72. Piccinni P, Dan M, Barbacini S, *et al.* Early isovolemic hemofiltration in oliguric patients with septic shock. *Intensive Care Med* 2006;32:80–6.

73. Bouman CS, Oudemans-Van Straaten HM, Tijssen JG, *et al.* Effects of early high-volume continuous venovenous hemofiltration on survival and recovery of renal function in intensive care patients with acute renal failure: A prospective, randomized trial. *Crit Care Med* 2002;30(10):2205–11.

74. Constantine J Karvellas, Maha R Farhat, Imran Sajjad, *et al.* A comparison of early versus late initiation of renal replacement therapy in critically ill patients with acute kidney injury: a systematic review and meta-analysis. *Critical Care* 2011;15:R72.

75. PICARD Group. Fluid accumulation, survival and recovery of kidney function in critically ill patients with acute kidney injury. *Kidney Intl* 2009;76:422–7.

76. Fulop T, Pathak MB, Schmidt DW, *et al.* Volume-related weight gain and subsequent mortality in acute renal failure patients treated with continuous renal replacement therapy. *ASAIO J* 2010;56(4):333–7.

Pitfall No. 4

Chasing the Wrong Target

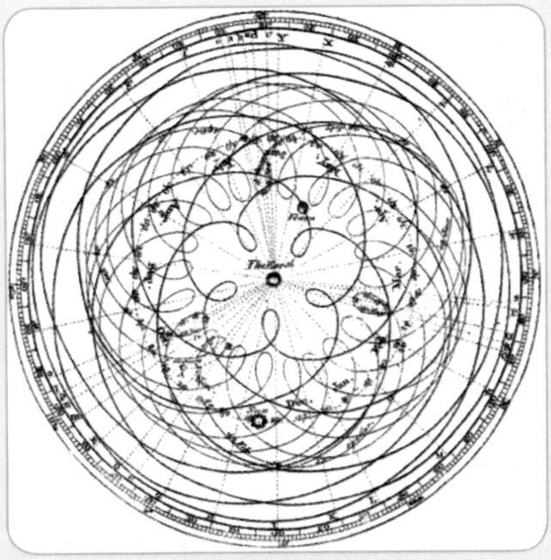

Physiological-Outcome Based Treatment

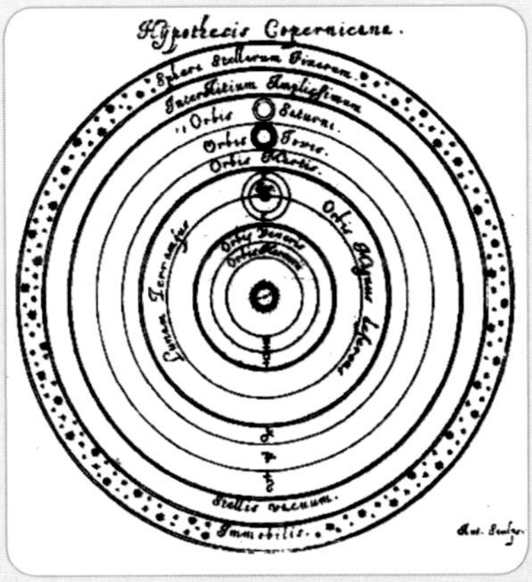

Clinical-Outcome Based Treatment

Figure 1. Comparison of the Ptolemaic and Copernican models of the solar system.

Pitfall No. 4

Choosing the Wrong Therapeutic Target

The pitfall is targeting a physiological or a surrogate outcome rather than a clinical one.

"The scientist is not a person who gives the right answers; he is one who asks the right questions."

– Claude Lévi-Strauss. French philosopher

In critical care

The Right Question is: which therapies improve clinical outcomes.

The Wrong Question is: which therapies improve physiological parameters.

Academicians and scientists are taught to think logically and base their concepts on plausible mechanisms. Based on these thoughts, one comes up with an idea or a guess, officially called a hypothesis. Then one makes a series of predictions based on what one would observe if these predictions were true. The next step is to design an experiment to test the hypothesis and see if the predictions occur as anticipated. If they do, one concludes that the hypothesis was correct. An initial hypothesis, through a positive experiment, has now become a conclusion. However, there is another way of doing science. Just see what works (predictions match outcomes) regardless of what the underlying mechanism is. This is a perfectly valid way of doing science. When Oliver Wendell Holmes and Semmelweis noted that hand washing decreased mortality, the germ theory of disease did not exist, yet their technique worked. Similarly though, we still do not know the nature or mechanism of consciousness, we know general anesthesia predictably and reliably suppresses it. Physicians, such as other scientists, tend to think of therapies through physiological mechanisms, and then do clinical trials for physiological or clinical outcomes. But all too

It is easier for clinicians to see the immediate physiological response to specific treatments than to gauge their impact on longer-term clinical outcomes like mortality and length of stay.

often, they accept that if an intervention changes the physiology for the better, then it must also improve outcome. Also, most physicians are reluctant to accept treatments that do not seem to be consistent with physiological concepts. These often result in physicians making errors of chasing the wrong targets or ignoring potentially useful therapies.

In some ways, it is stating the obvious that for intensive care patients and their relatives, the ONLY targets are improved clinical outcomes. But for clinicians, knowing which decisions favorably improve clinical outcomes is not as straight forward. As an example, clinicians routinely make decisions about starting a specific inotrope, starting renal replacement therapy (RRT) or changing antibiotics. It is very easy to see the physiological response to these treatments. One can see the blood pressure (BP) response to inotropes, the reversal of hyperkalemia with dialysis and the resolution of fever and leukocytosis with antibiotics. On the other hand, it is more difficult to clinically know how these decisions will impact longer-term outcomes such as length of stay, long-term morbidity and mortality. Because, it is easier to track the surrogates than actual clinical outcomes, they disproportionately influence bedside decision-making. It appears logical and plausible to presume that reversal of hypotension, hyperkalemia and fever will improve clinical outcomes. Unfortunately, studies have shown that many therapies successfully achieve their physiological target but do not impact outcome. In a significant number of studies the outcomes were worse. This is the intensive care unit (ICU) equivalent of "the operation was successful but the patient died."

This chapter focuses on how clinicians can be and have been misled by focusing on physiological surrogates rather than clinical outcomes.

Clinical Outcomes

Patients and families always desire positive outcomes as do the medical and nursing staff. The best outcome in ICU is reduced mortality which is fairly clear cut. But it isn't just mortality that needs to be reduced on ICU. Use of therapies and interventions that reduce morbidity and improve quality of life (QoL) are preferable to those that do not, even if they have similar mortality. Patient outcomes are also measured in terms of ventilator days, need and use of therapies such as RRT and vasoactive agents. Length of stay (LOS) is another useful clinical endpoint. This could be ICU LOS or hospital LOS. Obviously therapies with equal mortality but shorter ICU and hospital LOS are preferable to those with longer LOS.

Quality of Life scores and more recently, degree of functional rehabilitation are being used to evaluate therapies used on ICU. Health related QoL, as defined by the World Health Organization (WHO), is a subjective multidimensional state encompassing complete physical, mental and social wellbeing. It is a state that most survivors of critical illness will struggle to achieve unless structured interventions are in place. Given the added financial impact of poor physical recovery for patients, due to loss of earning capabilities depending on their pre-admission state, there is increasing interest in developing strategies aiming to emphasize functional rehabilitation to improve QoL.

This is further discussed in detail in Chapter 11 (Pitfall 9).

Surrogate or Physiological Outcomes

Monitoring and targeting physiological markers is one of the foundations of intensive care. We routinely measure and manipulate BP, central venous pressure (CVP), PaO_2, SaO_2, urine output and biochemical parameters. This is based on the plausible assumption that correction of these deranged parameters is beneficial to the patient. In itself, this is not a pitfall in the practice of critical care. *It becomes a pitfall when we assume that the correction of these factors will **unquestionably** lead to better **clinical** outcomes.* Once that assumption is made, the focus moves away from clinical to surrogate outcomes. The pitfall is the act of not questioning the impact of improved physiology on clinical outcome. If a series of studies had shown that this assumption was correct, then, this would be a simple way of practicing critical care. All we would be required to do would be to identify which physiological parameters are associated with improved clinical outcomes and target those. Unfortunately, a vast number of studies have shown that correcting physiology in critically ill patients does not translate into improved clinical outcomes. A simple example is the hydroxyethyl starch (HES) saga wherein the physiological markers such as circulating volume improved yet renal failure and mortality increased.

Intensive care patients and their relatives are looking for optimal clinical outcomes, not for sophisticated or hi-tech physiological manipulations.

Care of the critically ill individual is full of conflicting decisions.

Chasing physiological surrogates additionally brings its own set of problems, because each therapeutic intervention is aimed at a specific surrogate outcome. Often a therapy that improves one surrogate outcome will result in another physiological problem. The commonest one being that more fluids will preserve renal function and improve urine output, but worsen pulmonary function by precipitating pulmonary edema and over diuresing or drying out the patient can cure pulmonary edema but worsen azotemia.

Care of the critically ill individual is full of these kinds of decisions, and often the decision is made on the desires of the primary consultant, or the one who can make his or her case forcefully, rather than on the evidence of improved clinical outcomes. Equally often, different decisions made by various consultants are not aligned to the same goals and the overall treatment soon resembles a pastiche or a veritable smorgasbord, aimed less at patient outcome and more at prevention of conflict between various clinicians. The best thing clinicians can do in such a situation is to take a step back and figure out the correct questions which need to be tackled in treating the patients. At this point being primarily guided by high quality evidence based medicine (EBM) would be in the best interest of the patient as well as the team treating the patient. In this context, high quality EBM refers to large randomized controlled trials (RCTs) or meta-analysis of these RCTs, targeting clinical outcomes. Thus, the simplest way for clinicians to align decisions is to follow EBM and above all ask the appropriate questions. Once the questions are clearly defined, the management becomes much more streamlined. *And the right question is; will this therapy decrease mortality, and severity of illness, and will it speed up recovery and rehabilitation.*

A useful analogy of physiology based treatment versus outcome based treatment is comparing the models of the solar system (Figure 1). In an earlier era, the initial presumption was that the earth was at the centre and other bodies revolved around it. Creating a model that explained the observations became extremely convoluted and the version of Ptolemy was viewed as the most reliable, with its multiple "epicycles."

By simply changing one assumption, that the sun not the earth was in the centre, the newer Copernican model elegantly explained all the observations without the need of a series of complicated sub-orbits and epicycles. Patient care based on physiology alone leads to a similar Ptolemaic maze of conflicting decisions, while basing it on targeting clinical outcomes brings a Copernican elegance to practice. The only thing that really counts is a decrease in severity of disease, mortality and a quick and complete recovery. It would be best to view correction of physiology as a tool and improvements in clinical outcomes as a goal. The pitfall is not recognizing that correcting physiology alone isn't enough to improve clinical outcomes.

Evidence

Nitric Oxide (NO) is the physiological vasodilator in the body and its dysregulation in sepsis is believed to contribute to the shock state. It was therefore, physiologically plausible and sensible to inhibit it in septic shock. The use of the NO synthase inhibitor NG-methyl-L-arginine hydrochloride (546C88) was first studied in an RCT with the endpoint being resolution of shock (ref in Table 1) and shown to promote the resolution of shock with an acceptable safety profile. One would presume it was a good therapeutic option. Another RCT in the same year and the same journal studied the same molecule in the same setting, septic shock and found that there was a higher 28 day mortality (59 vs. 49% $P<0.01$). In fact, the trial was stopped early after review by the independent data safety monitoring board. This example really highlights the problem of asking the wrong question. If we ask the question; is this drug effective in the resolution of shock? The answer will be; it is effective and safe. Hence, it would be one more vasoactive drug added to our armamentarium. If we ask the question; does it improve mortality? The answer would be; no, it worsens it. It should therefore, be viewed as a poison and withdrawn from clinical use.

The story of intensivists chasing plausible pathophysiology and harming patients is shown in Table 1, where a series of interventions resulted in greater mortality of their patients. This approach is not limited to critical care. Table 2 shows similar disasters in mainstream medicine and surgery. Each time the drug did exactly what it was supposed to do and each time it increased mortality. It is worth stressing, that these are individual trials and later trials and meta-analysis may show a different outcome. The point of these two tables is to highlight the fact that one can achieve a physiological goal and yet harm the patient.

Correction of physiology is the tool, improvement in clinical outcomes is the goal.

Table 1. Intensive Care Trials with improved physiology or surrogates outcomes but worse clinical outcomes.

Therapy	Physiological target	Clinical outcome	Reference
HES	Circulating volume (compared to crystalloids)	Increased 90 day mortality Increased ARF requiring RRT	6S - N Engl J Med 2012, 367:124-134
HES	Circulating volume (compared to crystalloids)	Increased ARF requiring RRT	CHEST- N Engl J Med 2012; 367:1901-1911
Surgical ICP control	Decreased ICP in Traumatic brain injury	Worse neurological outcomes (Unfavourable score of 1-4 on Extended Glasgow Outcome Scale	DECRA - N Engl J Med 2011; 364:1493-1502
HFOV	Limit lung injury	Higher In-Hosp Mortality (Study stopped early on recommendation of the data monitoring committee)	OSCILLATE - N Engl J Med 2013;368:795
Insulin	Tight Sugar Control	Increased 90 day mortality	NICE-N Engl J Med 2009;360:1283-97
IV Fluid Bolus (pediatric population)	Volume resuscitation	Increased 48 hour mortality (Data and safety monitoring committee recommended halting recruitment)	FEAST- N Engl J Med 2011; 364:2483-2495
Early TPN	Nutrition	More infections, mechanical ventilation and RRT	N Engl J Med 2011; 365:506-17
Glutamine	Immuno Nutrition	Increased in-hospital and 6 month mortality	N Engl J Med 2013;368:1489-97
Growth Hormone	Promote Anabolism	Increased in hospital mortality	Takala. N Engl J Med 1999;341:785-92
Steroids in Sepsis	Immune modulation	Increased 14 day mortality in subgroup with raised creatinine	Bone 1987 N Engl J Med.1987 Sep 10;317(11):653-8.
Nitric Oxide synthase inhibitor NG-methyl-L-arginine hydrochloride (546C88)	Resolution of shock	Increased 28 day mortality (Stopped early by independent data safety monitoring board)	Bakker. Crit Care Med 2004; 32:1–12 and Lopez. Crit Care Med 2004; 32:21–30

Table 2. Medical and surgical therapies that corrected pathophysiological parameters but increased mortality

Therapy	Surrogate endpoint	Patient endpoint	Reference
Encainide and Flecainide	Decreased dysrhythmias	Increased mortality	CAST 1-Echt DS, *et al.* N Engl J Med. 1991 Mar 21;324(12):781-8.
Moricizine	Decreased dysrhythmias	Increased mortality	CAST II. N Engl J Med. 1992;327:227-233
Lignocaine	Decreased VF	Increased mortality	Arch Intern Med. 1989 Dec;149(12):2694-8
Dronedarone	Rate control for Atrial Fibrillation	Increased mortality	PALLAS Investigators N Engl J Med 2011; 365:2268-2276
Milrinone	Increased cardiac contractility	Increased mortality	Packer M, *et al.* N Engl J Med. 1991 Nov 21;325(21):1468-75.
Ibopamine	Increased cardiac contractility	Increased mortality	Hampton JR, *et al.* Lancet.1997 Apr 5;349(9057):971-7.
Epoprostenol	Increased cardiac contractility	Increased mortality	Califf RM, *et al.* Am Heart J. 1997 Jul;134(1):44-54.
Nesiritide	Decreased wedge pressure	Increased mortality	Sackner-Bernstein JD, *et al. JAMA* 2005 Apr 20;293(15):1900-5.
Doxazosin	Decreased blood pressure	Increased mortality	Messerli FH, *et al.* Curr Hypertens Rep. 2000 Jun;2(3):241-2.
Torcetrapib	Decreased cholesterol	Increased mortality	Barter PJ, *et al.* N Engl J Med. 2007 Nov 22;357(21):2109-22.
Phenformin	Decreased blood sugar	Increased mortality	University Group Diabetes Program. Diabetes. 1975;24 Suppl 1:65–184.
Erythropoietin	Increased hemoglobin in renal failure	Increased mortality	Phrommintikul A, *et al.* Lancet. 2007 Feb;369(9559):381–388.
Aprotinin	Decreased blood loss in cardiac surgery	Increased mortality	Fergusson DA, *et al.* N Engl J Med. 2008 May;358(22):2319–2331.
Metoprolol	Decreased perioperative ischemia	Increased mortality	Devereaux PJ, *et al.* Lancet. 2008 May;371(9627):1839–1847.

Conclusion

It is important to maintain focus on clinical outcomes rather than surrogate ones. It is relatively easy to target and monitor physiology and presume that this is improving clinical outcomes, but this is often not the case. Clinicians must be aware of the literature which demonstrates which physiological targets result in better clinical outcomes and which ones do not. One could then limit therapy to those that improve both surrogate and clinical outcomes.

Pitfall No. 5

Less is More

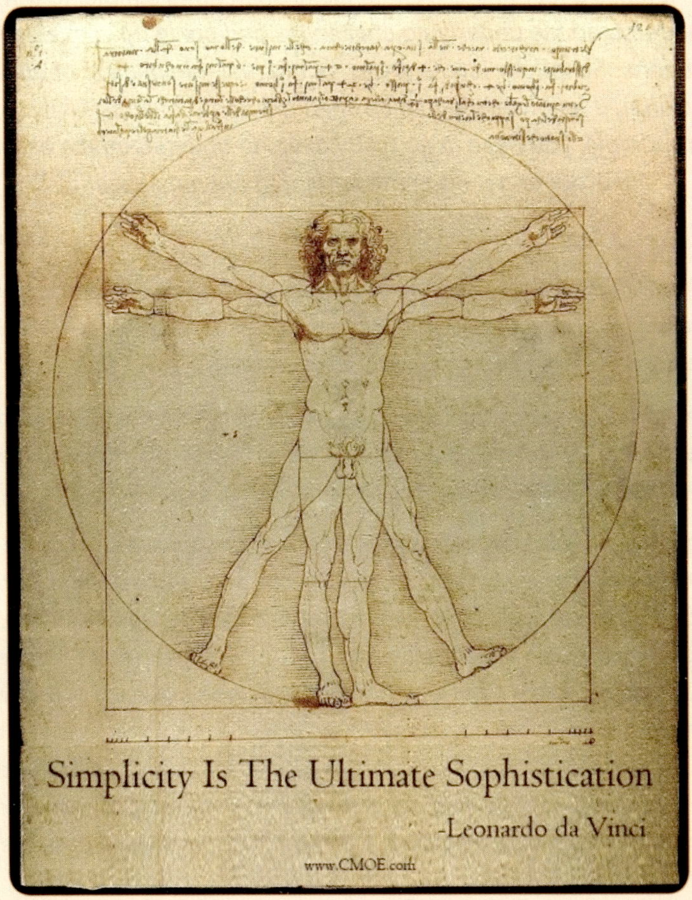

Pitfall No. 5

Doing Too Much: Can Less Be More?

"It takes a lot of hard work to make something simple, to truly understand the underlying challenges and come up with elegant solutions. Simplicity isn't a style. It's not just minimalism or absence of clutter. It involves digging through the depth of complexity. To be truly simple, you have to go really deep, to understand the essence in order to get rid of the parts that are not essential."

– Steve Jobs

This chapter aims at digging deep into the literature to understand the essence (improving clinical outcomes) in order to get rid of the parts that are not essential (therapies that are ineffective or that improve surrogate but not clinical outcomes).

The intensive care community is increasingly exploring this question. It is usually put forward as a statement, "Less is More", i.e. by doing less we can have better outcomes. It is better to currently ask, can less be more?, rather than simply state it.

This particular chapter is the most speculative of all the potential pitfalls covered in the book. It is better viewed as a hypothesis. The question being: Will a Liberal versus Restrictive approach to therapies result in better clinical outcomes in intensive care patients. The Liberal Approach involves using all the proven therapies and using all other plausible therapies that have not yet been demonstrated to be effective. The Restrictive approach involves limiting the therapies to proven ones, and selectively and judiciously using other techniques based on clinical evaluation of the individual patient. Needless to say it is desirable for practitioners of both approaches to avoid using disproved therapies, solely based on their experience and historical data. In some ways, this is already happening, for example, most ICUs have

If two therapies result in the same clinical outcomes, it makes no sense to use the costlier or more complicated one.

now stopped "routinely" changing vascular catheters and indwelling tubes, though this was considered standard practice in the early era of intensive care. Similarly, there has been a decrease in the frequency of routine investigations such as arterial blood gases and chest X-rays in ventilated patients.

This chapter will cover, selectively, literature in which adding on additional therapies has resulted in no improvement or even patient harm. Obviously there will be some countering literature, some of it not covered in the chapter. So, it could be viewed as one part of a pro-con debate, supporting a restrictive approach. The primary aim is not to suggest that one should always be restrictive, but to be aware of the limitations and potential harms of being liberal and offering every possible therapy to all ICU patients. The main argument against doing too much is that there are clinical adverse outcomes noted with many therapies and these can be minimized by only using treatments proven to improve clinical outcomes.

There is a second non-clinical argument, that of preventing resources from unnecessarily being spent. If two therapies result in the same clinical outcomes, it makes no sense to use the costlier or more complicated one. For example, multiple studies have shown that targeting a hemoglobin (Hb) of > 7 is associated with the same clinical outcomes as targeting a Hb > 9-10. If this is true, it makes no sense to transfuse blood purely on the basis of an Hb of between 7 and 10. It adds to expense and does not help the patient in any way. Another example would be the use of either intravenous Immunoglobulins (IVIg) or plasmapheresis (PP) in Guillain Barre Syndrome (GBS). Combining the two has not been shown to improve recovery or outcome, compared to either one alone. If the patient does not respond to one, it is cheaper and easier to wait for recovery to occur, rather than add the second treatment. This could be viewed as a variation of 'Occam's Razor' that has been stated in many forms. The most relevant version, from a scientific perspective, is "when you have two competing theories that make exactly the same predictions, the simpler one is the better." This "Law of Parsimony" could be equally applied to therapeutics. "When you have two competing therapies that give exactly the same clinical outcomes, the simpler and cheaper one is the better." Put another way, if less is equal, then less is more; equal in terms of clinical outcomes but more in terms of savings in financial and professional resources.

Unfortunately, the financial incentive can work both ways. Pharmaceutical companies would obviously want to increase sales, and would do what is needed in making the medical community prescribe their products. But there are also hospital based incentives. The more drugs and devices used, the more the hospital can earn by adding their costs. Similarly, the more investigations, the more the hospital earns. And finally medical professionals are also incentivized in terms of payments by doing more procedures. Medical professionals have their "performances" evaluated by hospital administrators, a laudable idea. All too often the performance is not related to the patient outcomes but the "volume of business" generated. This actually puts pressure on clinicians to do some things they do not actually believe are beneficial. In situations where therapies are clearly useful, or useless, one can follow the data and practice appropriately. But a large number of treatments have minimal effect, and in those circumstances, many clinicians will feel pressurized to do them to "keep up the numbers."

It is difficult to get a man to understand something, when his salary depends on his not understanding it.

– Upton Sinclair

This is no longer an academic question. It is being increasingly pointed out by the medical community in their journals[1] and in the lay press[2,3] that vast medical resources are being wasted by routinely doing large numbers of ineffective investigations and procedures.

It is easier to do something than to do nothing, and the pressure to do something is much more in the context of an ICU patient than a stable patient on the ward or in outpatient clinics. In response, investigations and therapies are added just to demonstrate that "everything possible is being done." In essence this is no different to a witch doctor performing an elaborate ritual to convince the "customer/client/patient" that he or she is actually doing something useful. A more charitable way of looking at this approach of "do everything" is that it is a skillful use of the placebo effect. The placebo effect is very real and can offer significant improved outcomes for patients, usually for neuro-cognitive symptoms. In the ICU context, this placebo effect is really more for the relatives, as the patient often is not lucid enough. We will present the data behind many of the current therapies used in ICU and acute medicine

Vast medical resources are being wasted by routinely doing large numbers of ineffective investigations and procedures.

Growth hormone may enhance performance in athletes, but it doubled mortality in critically ill.

and let the reader decide if they are effective treatments, evolving treatments or ineffective rituals.

"Don't just do something, Stand there"

– The White Rabbit (from the film Alice in Wonderland)

Evidence

Before we cover each standard ICU or medical –surgical therapy that can potentially cause harm, we would like to start with 4 illustrative examples.

In the 19th century, there was a cholera epidemic in London.[4] At that time, there was no proven treatment for cholera. Some patients were admitted to the Middlesex (Allopathic) Hospital while others went to the London Homeopathy Hospital. A series of studies[5] have now shown that homeopathy is no better than placebo. So, we could view this as an observational study comparing two cohorts receiving different forms of treatment, with the allopathic hospital group being the treatment arm and the homeopathic group being the placebo controlled arm. Mortality at London Homeopathy Hospital was ~30% that at Middlesex (Allopathic) Hospital. It appears that the act of giving allopathic medicine and using other techniques such as "blood letting" were not only ineffective, they were dangerous. So dangerous, that the placebo patients had just one-third the mortality compared to those admitted to the allopathic hospital.

If the first example of medical therapies causing harm is historical, the second should be viewed as a modern cautionary ICU tale. Growth Hormone (GH) is known to promote anabolism and tissue buildup, so it was perfectly plausible to assume it would speed up recovery in critically ill. Takala and colleagues[6] studied this in a concurrent two-arm trial. There were minor differences in the way the two concurrent arms were managed. In effect this could be viewed as 2 parallel RCTs. The trial was well conducted, it was double blind, placebo controlled and looked at a meaningful endpoint i.e. mortality. The findings were troubling, to say the least. There was essentially a doubling of mortality because of the use of growth hormone. In the Finnish arm of the study, the GH versus control mortality was 39% vs, 20% and in the multi-national arm of the study it was 44% vs. 18%. Among those who survived, those who received GH had longer durations of mechanical ventilation, and increased length of stay (LOS) in ICU. This is a very useful example when evaluating whether one should use a therapy that is plausible but untested to clinical outcomes. If this study had not been done, many practitioners would have continued to use GH with the presumption that the increased anabolism would improve the patients' recovery. A liberal approach to using untested therapies would have harmed patients while a restrictive one would have resulted in a lower mortality.

The third example where doing more in an ICU can be counterproductive is in relation to patients with a terminal disease, in this particular case, metastatic non–small cell lung cancer. Traditionally patients are referred to a palliative care physician or service in the late stages of their illness. In this study,[(7)] early in the disease, a few weeks after diagnosis of metastatic non-small cell lung cancer patients were enrolled and randomized to early palliation or standard care. The aim was to see if the early introduction of palliative care helped quality of life. Not surprisingly it did. Part of the palliative care management was the documentation of preferences for aggressive care and ICU at the end of life. More patients in the early palliative care group had documented their preferences than those in the standard care group. What was surprising was that though more patients in the standard treatment group received aggressive ICU care than those in the palliative care group, the median survival was higher in those receiving palliative care and less ICU therapy. One should be cautious of reading too much into this. This trial was not designed to primarily see the effect of offering aggressive end of life ICU care on length of subsequent survival. But, it is surprising that those patients receiving intensive care should have a shorter survival. As it was a randomized trial, it is not that sicker patients went to ICU and hence, there was a bias towards early mortality. A popular medical author has described this as "almost Zen like". The less one focused on living long, the longer one ended up living. A more pragmatic interpretation was that aggressive intensive care, caused immediate physiological stabilization, but resulted in a series of complications that resulted in a higher subsequent mortality.

This last example appeared in a section titled "Less is More" in JAMA.[8] It is an interesting observational trial that looked at the 30 day mortality of more than 200,000 cardiology patient admissions over a decade. They compared outcomes of those admitted during major cardiology conferences to periods preceding and following the meeting. During conferences, presumably many senior cardiologist would be away and there would be less expert personnel than during non-conference periods. They noted that patients with acute

Some ICU therapies that have been used routinely and unquestioningly for decades may be worthless and even potentially dangerous.

myocardial infarction (MI) admitted during the conference periods got less intervention in terms of Percutaneous Coronary Interventions (PCI) but had similar mortality to those admitted in the non-conference periods. Surprisingly, they noted that patients admitted as emergencies with cardiac failure and those who had a cardiac arrest actually had a lower mortality during these periods when cardiologists were away at the conference. One should not read too much into this observational data, but at the least it should raise the question; can we lower mortality in cardiac patients by doing less.

Can Less be More?

Standard ICU Therapies

We briefly review some literature regarding standard ICU therapies and highlight that using them routinely and unquestioningly may be worthless, or even dangerous. We look at Oxygen therapy, adrenaline and ACLS in CPR, blood products, nutrition, sugar control, steroids and DVT prophylaxis. We also briefly look at the impact of some investigational techniques such as CT scans.

Oxygen Therapy

Oxygen is often believed to be "the breath of life" and history and cult behind it are so strong, that it is routinely and unquestioningly used in almost all sick patients. To some extent, this is a historical anomaly. Oxygen was cheaply and widely available well before pulse oximetry. And since, mild hypoxemia could not be detected clinically; it made sense to use it liberally in anyone who might be marginally hypoxemic. In contemporary ICUs, pulse oximetry is ubiquitous and there is really no reason to use oxygen among patients with oxygen saturations above 90%. Implementing this alone may result is meaningful cost savings. But, oxygen may actually be harmful if used liberally. A recent review[9] highlighted literature from the last few decades suggesting oxygen may not be safe in many clinical circumstances (Table 1). Most of these however are based on surrogate outcomes.

Table 1. Effects of Supplemental Oxygen in Different Clinical Conditions[9]

Clinical Condition	Effect Parameter	Effect	Reference
Exercise testing	ECG alterations	Prolonged	*JAMA.* 1950;144:373-375
Post myocardial infarction	Heart rate	Decreased	*Lancet.* 1964;2(7364):825-832
	Stroke volume	Decreased	*Br Heart J.* 1965;27:401-407
	Cardiac output	Decreased	*Br Med J.* 1968;4(5627):360-364
	Systemic vascular resistance	Increased	
	Mean arterial pressure	Increased	
Acute myocardial infarction	Vascular resistance of LAD	Increased	*J Appl Physiol.* 2007;102(5):2040-2045
Cardiac catheterization	Coronary vascular resistance	Increased	*Am J Physiol.* 2005;288(3):H1057-H1062
	Coronary blood flow	Decreased	
Congestive heart failure	Stroke volume	Decreased	*J Am Coll Cardiol.* 1996;27(2):353-357
	Heart rate	Decreased	*Am J Physiol Heart Circ Physiol.* 2002;282(6):H2414-2421
	Cardiac output	Decreased	*Chest.* 2001;120(2):467-473
	Systemic vascular resistance	Increased	*Heart.* 2010;96(7):533-538
	LV end diastolic pressure	Increased	
	Isovolumetric relaxation time	Increased	
COPD	Hypercapnia	Increased	*Clin Med.* 2002;2(5):449-451
	Mortality	Increased	*BMJ.* 2010;341:c5462
Stroke	Stroke severity score	Increased	*Stroke.* 2003;34(2):571-574
	Mortality	Increased	*Stroke.* 1999;30(10):2033 – 2037 NCT00414726[a]
Cardiopulmonary resuscitation	Neuron-specific enolase	Elevated	*Resuscitation.* 2006:69(2);199-206
	Mortality	Increased	*JAMA.* 2010;303(21):2165-2171
			Circulation. 2011;123(23):2717-2722
			Critical Care. 2011;15(2):R90

Abbreviations: COPD, chronic obstructive pulmonary disease; ECG, electrocardiogram; LAD, left anterior descending coronary artery; LV, left ventricular.
[a]Trial was terminated (Clinical Trial of Normobaric Oxygen Therapy in Acute Ischemic Stroke, not published, clinicaltrials.gov Identifier: NCT00414726).

Excess oxygen increased mortality or morbidity in COPD, AMI & CPR.

A large observational study looked at clinical outcomes following cardiopulmonary resuscitation (CPR).[10] They tested the hypothesis that post-resuscitation hyperoxia is associated with increased mortality. They defined hyperoxia as being > 300mmHg/40 kPa, and hypoxemia as being < 60 mmHg/8 kPa. They found that among patients admitted to the ICU following resuscitation from cardiac arrest, arterial hyperoxia was independently associated with increased in-hospital mortality compared with either hypoxia or normoxia. In other words, not only did the patients who had a PaO_2 > 300 mmHg/40 kPa do worse than those with a normal oxygen level, they also did worse than patients who were hypoxemic. Though this is an observational study, it should caution against the liberal use of oxygen, at least in those with a vulnerable brain, following a central nervous system (CNS) insult.

A recent RCT looked at a liberal versus restrictive use of oxygen therapy in acute exacerbation of COPD (AECOPD) in the pre hospital phase of the illness.[11] They compared oxygen delivered at a higher flow rate of 8-10 lpm via face mask against a low flow nasal cannula targeting a SaO_2 of 88-92%.They found that the risk of death in all patients with suspected AECOPD was significantly reduced by 58% with titrated oxygen treatment. In the subgroup of patients with confirmed COPD, the risk of death was reduced by 78% with titrated oxygen treatment.

A recent paper regarding O_2 in acute myocardial infarction threw up some interesting findings. The Air Versus Oxygen in Myocardial Infarction (AVOID)[12] study was a randomized multicenter trial of 441 non-hypoxemic (SaO2 >93%) patients with confirmed ST elevation myocardial infarction (STEMI). They looked at surrogate and clinical end points. The use of oxygen in these patients was associated with higher rates of arrhythmias and recurrent myocardial infarctions. It was also associated with larger initial infarct size as judged by CK-MB and Troponin peak and also larger infarct size at 6 months as evaluated by cardiac MR.

If one puts the information from the earlier review and both the above recent trials, it appears that a restrictive use of oxygen is safer than a liberal one. This is especially true in the current era of universal SaO_2 monitoring. If there is a role for liberal oxygen, it would be in brain injured patients without SaO_2 monitoring where even a minor degree of hypoxemia results in worse neurological outcomes.

Cardio-Pulmonary Resuscitation (CPR)

Cardio-Pulmonary Resuscitation techniques have evolved over the last 5-6 decades. Most of these were discarding of medicines and techniques which were ineffective. Intra cardiac injections now appear quaint, and lignocaine, bicarbonate and calcium are no longer routinely used in CPR. Contemporary CPR is based around Basic Life Support (BLS) and Advanced Life Support (ALS). Basic Life Support too has been simplified to chest compressions with little or no interruption for artificial ventilation.[13, 14] The real advance in CPR was rapid electrical defibrillation for Ventricular Fibrillation or Pulseless ventricular tachycardia (VT-VF). In fact this became considered as part of BLS, and then automated external devices (AEDs) were shown to be beneficial when used by paramedics and lay public.[15,16] Disappointingly the use of AEDs, in hospital did not improve outcomes, and actually worsened them is some settings.[17]

Advanced Life Support (ALS) consists of the use of devices and drugs in addition to BLS. Studies in the last decade have made us question some of our basic assumptions about the effectiveness of ALS. A study also looked at the impact of using airway devices instead of simple bag mask ventilation and found that the use of these devices was associated with worse neurological outcomes.[18]

One could speculate that any time lost from chest compression during BLS worsens outcomes by compromising chest compressions and cardio-cerebral perfusion during BLS. Attempts at finding venous access, delivering drugs or waiting for AEDs to analyse rhythms could potentially decrease the efficacy of BLS.

After rapid cardioversion intravenous adrenaline is currently the mainstay of ALS. It is worth following the evolution of this seemingly effective treatment.

Adrenaline in CPR

In 1963, John W Pearson and Joseph S Redding published a thoughtful paper on adrenaline in CPR.[19] They noted that people had mentioned the use of adrenaline sporadically for 15 years, but there was no consensus on how it should be used. They speculated on whether the beneficial effect was cardiac or on the peripheral circulation. They felt it should be given intracardiac as intravenous would result in delay of action. They noted that a dose of 1 mg (1 mL of a 1 in 1000 solution) could be excessively high. They cite a paper which suggested 5 mL of this solution and speculate if that was a printing error!! Papers like this set the widespread use of adrenaline in all forms of shockable and non-shockable CPR. Intracardiac adrenaline use fell over a period of time, but adrenaline remained the mainstay of treatment.

Adrenaline may be ineffective in CPR.

Over half a century, the role of adrenaline in CPR became more entrenched. Three well conducted studies in the 1990s found that high-dose (5 mg) was not superior to standard dose (1 mg) adrenaline.[20-22]

Cardio-Pulmonary Resuscitation is the ultimate emergency, and hence, presents the biggest hurdles to research. In the context of a trial for an immediately life threatening situation, it is difficult to suggest that control patients should not get the treatment, or only get placebo. For practical purposes, consent cannot be taken from either patient or relative prior to enrolling, and since, more than 90% do not survive, it is difficult to know what to tell relatives, if the patient had been enrolled in a trial (on presumptive consent) and then did not survive.

After more than half a century of unquestioning use, in the last 5-6 years, there have been a series of studies which make us question if it works at all. The first study to raise doubt about efficacy was the PACA (Placebo versus Adrenaline in Cardiac Arrest) trial.[23] This was a placebo controlled RCT in the pre hospital setting. The authors concluded that hospital discharge (primary endpoint) was similar and ROSC (secondary endpoint) was more in the study group, leaving the interpretation open to the reader. Even though adrenaline did not decrease mortality, the authors appeared reluctant to expressly state that it was ineffective. They implied it is probably effective and the uncertainty may be more related to the trial than to the drug itself. Amazingly, the editorial to this negative trial was titled, "Adrenaline-Proven benefit in cardiac arrest at last?".[24]

This "proven benefit" was increased ROSC, and the authors implied that the study was underpowered for mortality. There is a back-story to why the trial was underpowered, and it serves as a useful parable of the power of tradition over science. Many potential participants, mostly ambulance paramedics, felt it was "unethical" to withhold adrenaline in cardiac arrest because they "knew" that it worked. To make matters more complicated, these people took their objection to the lay press and loudly proclaimed that the investigators were experimenting with patients' lives. As a result, many states in Australia did not participate in the study. The participation could be summarized by the following sentence. The state that did not use adrenaline routinely in pre hospital CPR agreed to participate, while the states that did use it refused to participate.

Interestingly, there actually was earlier data from 2009 in a prospective RCT suggesting that adrenaline may be ineffective.[25] In this study, the controls got no venous catheter or IV medication and the outcome was similar. The authors in 2012 then did a post hoc analysis of the same data for the adrenaline effect and found that adrenaline did not improve long-term mortality.[26]

The lead authors of both these studies unfortunately faced a lot of hostility from lay and medical public before the results came out and seriously questioned the efficacy of adrenaline in out of hospital CPR.

Since, then there have been a series of observational trials and meta-analysis questioning the efficacy of adrenaline in CPR, but it continues to be a part of the guidelines. This problem with guidelines not adapting to literature will be further explored in a later chapter. Most of this literature is based on out of hospital CPR, so one should be cautious of extrapolating it to in-hospital patients.[27 - 31]

So, where are we with adrenaline in CPR today? We no longer use it intra-cardiac, and 1 mg, rather than 5 mg, is the recommended dose. The guidelines continue to recommend it, and at present this is probably the right thing to do. However, this now must be seen as a recommendation based on weak and questionable evidence. It may be more appropriate for guidelines to state that they are unable to give a recommendation for the role of adrenaline in out of hospital CPR.

CPR and Hypothermia

In 2002, 2 trials showed neurological benefit by inducing hypothermia in survivors of out of hospital cardiac arrest.[32,33] Two recent studies (TTM[34] and THAPCA[35]) have not demonstrated a benefit of active cooling after CPR. In the former, called Targeted temperature Management (TTM), 33 vs. 36 degree Celcius was compared in adults, while the later was a pediatric trial. Regardless, it is prudent to prevent fever in the post resuscitation phase as this may be neuro protective.

Blood Transfusion

Historical convention was that it was appropriate to transfuse critically ill patients to keep the hemoglobin above 10 gm/dL (100 gm/L). In 1999, a large Canadian trial tested two targets, >7 gm/dL (restrictive group) and >10 gm/dL (liberal group) in 838 patients and found no

---

Targeted Temperature after cardiac arrest: Not too cool, not too warm.

Transfusing blood to ICU patients with hemoglobin of more than 7 gm/dL is a needless waste of precious blood.

impact on mortality or other relevant clinical outcomes.[36] They noted that younger patients with less severe illness had lower mortality in the restrictive group. At this point, it was suggested that the potential negative aspects of packed red blood cells (PRBC) transfusion may be due to the age of the PRBC, with older PRBCs occluding the microcirculation, or due to the presence of WBCs, with their known immune modulating effects. There was also a question of the relevance of this data to patients with ischemic heart disease. One investigator[37] did a retrospective study in acute myocardial infarction (AMI) in those more than 65 years old, from data of 78,974 Medicare beneficiaries. They noted an increase in 30 day mortality if HCT <30 and questionable benefit if HCT 30-33. This lead the Canadians to do a subgroup analysis[38] of 357 out of the 838 patients with CVS disease. They found no difference in mortality, no difference in CVS complications, but possible benefit in AMI and unstable Angina.

Two cohort studies, largely using leuco-depleted blood gave ambiguous results.[39, 40] Recently a large study (TRISS[41]) looked at the outcomes of a restrictive versus a liberal strategy. They compared outcomes in approximately 1000 patients randomized to receive leuco-depleted blood to maintain either a target of 7 or 9 gm/dL hemoglobin (Hb). They noted that the 90 day mortality, the incidence of ischemic events and the need for life support were similar in both groups. Another study (ABLE[42]) looked at the impact of age of the PRBC on clinical outcomes. Again, more than a 1000 patients were enrolled, and the treatment group got PRBC less than 8 days old while the control group got standard issue PRBC units. They noted no difference between the two groups in terms of primary outcome of 90 day mortality, or in terms of secondary outcomes (major illnesses, duration of respiratory, hemodynamic, or renal support, length of stay in the hospital, and transfusion reactions) or in the subgroup analyses.

This growing body of data strongly suggests that transfusing patients above a value of 7 gm/dL does not improve clinical outcome. This remains true if regular or leuco-depleted blood is used, and regardless of the duration of storage of the PRBCs. It is difficult to justify routine PRBC transfusions in ICU patients with a Hb of more than 7 gm/dL.

Nutrition

This is a topic on which the literature is not very clear. Physiologically energy is required during a critical illness, but there is a vast reserve of calories in terms of fat and protein in the body. In the context of starvation, people who go on hunger strike, or are lost in the wilderness have survived between 45-60 days on water alone. On one hand one could argue that early nutrition will limit catabolism of body tissue, but on the other hand one could argue that feeding, absorption and anabolism has its own metabolic costs and this could further overload the hyper metabolic state. As part of the early nutrition strategy, there was a trend to promote "post-pyloric" feeding with special tubes in the hope that enteral nutrition could be started earlier. The belief was that gastro-paresis is common in critically ill but the small bowel, retains peristalsis and hence, can be used earlier. The use of this has decreased over the last decade.

The main issues in nutrition are:

- Should nutrition be started early
- Is there an advantage in choosing enteral or parenteral
- Is there any role for immune enhancing or other organ specific feeds?

Early Enteral or Parenteral Nutrition

In 2011, the ESICM Systematic Review Group reviewed the critical care literature. They covered some aspects of nutrition.[43]

Regarding early nutrition (within 24 hours) they noted in a meta-analysis of 5 studies that there appeared to be a reduction in mortality and pneumonia associated with early enteral nutrition. The authors generally recommend early enteral nutrition but the experts noted that there was substantial clinical heterogeneity and felt one could not make robust and valid conclusions for a general ICU population.

A recent pragmatic RCT[44] looked at the effect of early enteral versus parenteral nutrition in close to 2500 patients with approximately half receiving enteral and the other half receiving parenteral nutrition. They found similar 30 day all cause mortality, infection rates and no difference in 14 other secondary endpoints. They noted a higher incidence of vomiting and hypoglycemia in the enteral group. Interestingly, in both groups they found that most patients did not meet their nutrition targets.

The EPaNIC trial,[45] was a large RCT of more than 2000 patients in whom half were randomized to early TPN (< 48 hours) and the others to late (> 8 days). All patients additionally got enteral nutrition as tolerated. The late TPN group had fewer infections and some marginal benefits in terms of need of mechanical ventilation, RRT and ICU-LOS. Not surprisingly costs were lower too. The overall mortality was same in both groups. There were some questions

Early enteral nutrition is probably useful while early parenteral nutrition may be harmful.

raised and these were addressed in a post hoc analysis of this paper which showed no indication that more severely ill patients benefit from early parenteral nutrition. The untoward effect of early enhanced nutrition is not restricted to patients receiving the highest energy doses. Also, a relatively high protein-to-glucose ratio is not associated with better outcome.[46]

The other TPN trial looked at the early use of TPN in more than 1300 patients with relative contraindications to early enteral nutrition.[47] The overall mortality was the same but the authors noted a shorter duration of ventilation and associated cost saving due to this.

Immunonutrition

Nutrition in ICU has taken another interesting direction in the last 1-2 decades. Conventionally nutrition is just that, calories, proteins, electrolytes, micro-nutrients such as vitamins and trace elements, delivered in an appropriate volume of water. A concept of "immune-nutrition" evolved, based on the concept that the gut, teeming with bacteria, was the great un-drained abscess of the body. This form of nutrition was designed to protect the vulnerable bowel wall by supplementing amino acids such as glutamine, arginine, taurine, glycine, as well as other pharmaconutrients such as some omega fatty acids, nucleotides, fibre and antioxidants. These were believed to also be immune modulating by limiting pro-inflammatory mediators and improving immune cellular function. Initial studies were promising and 2 meta-analysis[48, 49] and an RCT[50] showed promise in terms of less infection, mortality and LOS. This was followed by a series of trials which showed that the use of oral arginine and other nutrients either do not improve clinical outcomes or occasionally may worsen outcomes, especially in critically ill septic patients.[51] The focus then shifted to immune nutrition in perioperative rather than ICU patients and to the use of IV rather than enteral glutamine. Recently a large RCT looked at the use of IV glutamine and anti-oxidants in ICU patients[52] and found that anti-oxidants did not improve mortality while glutamine actually increased mortality.

Overall, it appears that it is advisable to start early enteral nutrition when the gut is working. But there is no rush to start TPN and starting too early may actually result in a more complicated ICU stay. Currently, there is no role for immune or pharma-nutrition.

Sugar Control

Glucose control in critically ill patients has been studied in some detail in the last 15-20 years. Furnary, a cardiac surgeon with a degree in biochemistry, demonstrated that normoglycemia was associated with lower surgical site infections[53] and mortality.[54] His data also suggested that IV insulin achieved this better than subcutaneous insulin, and it was the perioperative blood sugar per se, rather than the history of diabetes that determined the perioperative increase in infections and mortality. This was followed by the Van den Berg paper,[55] in high risk surgical patients where keeping the blood sugar in the normal range of 80-110 mg/dL was associated with decreased infection, mortality, length of ICU stay, renal dysfunction and critical illness neuropathy. This was labeled as intensive insulin therapy, and there were some questions as to whether the benefit was due to normoglycemia, or directly due to insulin. The next paper from the same group,[56] this time in medical ICU patients failed to show a mortality benefit, but the treatment group patients had lower LOS and less renal failure. This was followed by two trials, VISEP trial[57] and the European Glucontrol trial[58] which were halted prematurely because of a high incidence of hypoglycemia in the intensive insulin therapy group. Finally, a large study of more than 6000 patients was conducted by the ANZICS (Australia and New Zealand) group[59] and they found a higher all cause mortality in the intensive insulin treatment group. This was a surprising finding. Even more surprising was that the 28 day mortality was similar in both groups. It is difficult to interpret this. Why should insulin or normoglycemia during the ICU phase of the critical illness cause a delayed increase in mortality? Regardless, after this large trial with an adverse mortality outcome, intensive insulin therapy targeting normoglycemia is no longer recommended in critically ill patients.

DVT Prophylaxis

DVT prophylaxis in ICU and perioperative patients has reached cult status, and it is assumed that not taking appropriate measures is negligent. So, it is worth pointing out that all the positive studies have primarily looked at surrogate endpoints (detection of DVT). The creators of guidelines are unable to quote a single study which shows that clinical outcomes are improved by perioperative DVT prophylaxis and subsequently, not a single recommendation

The NICE study with more than 6000 patients found a higher all cause mortality in those treated with intensive Insulin Therapy targeting Normoglycemia.

Prophylaxis prevents Deep Vein Thrombosis, but no study has shown that this translates to Lower Mortality.

of the ACCP guidelines 9th Edition (Chest 2012) have a 1 A recommendation.[60] It doesn't help credibility when these guideline creations are supported by industry.

In acutely ill medical patients only one large RCT (LIFENOX)[61] has looked at the impact of Low Molecular Weight Heparin (LMWH) on clinical outcomes and found that it was similar among patients who did not receive LMWH. A study specific to ICU patients compared conventional heparin to LMWH and again found no difference in all major clinical outcomes.[62] One large analysis looked at multiple studies that included mortality data in orthopedic patients after hip or knee surgery. The primary aim was to see the impact of choice of DVT prophylaxis therapy on clinical endpoints, in this case pulmonary embolism and all cause mortality.[63] The studies included about 30,000 patients who were classified into three groups. Group A consisted of 15,839 patients receiving low-molecular-weight heparin, ximelagatran, fondaparinux, or rivaroxaban. Group B consisted of 7193 receiving regional anesthesia, pneumatic compression and aspirin and Group C had 5006 receiving warfarin. All-cause mortality was higher in Group A than in Group B (0.41% vs. 0.19%) and the incidence of clinical non-fatal pulmonary embolus was higher in Group A than in Group B (0.60% vs. 0.35%).The incidences of all-cause mortality and non-fatal pulmonary embolism in Group C were similar to those in Group A (0.4 and 0.52, respectively). The authors concluded that clinical pulmonary embolus occurs despite the use of anticoagulants and the use of potent anticoagulants was associated with the highest all-cause mortality of the three modalities studied.

Conclusion: There is an large body of data that suggests that pharmaceutical prophylaxis prevents DVTs as diagnosed on duplex sonography and doppler. But almost no study has shown that this translates to improved clinical outcomes.

Steroids

People Die. Steroids never do.

– Anonymous

Steroids have many beneficial effects and are potentially lifesaving in certain medical conditions such as asthma or autoimmune diseases. Many physicians believe that this benefit could also be seen in main stream ICU conditions. In the 1980s, the role of high-dose early steroids in ARDS and septic shock was studied and consistently found to be either ineffective or harmful (Table 2). These early high-dose regimes were slowly given up. Small studies looked at alternative regimes with variable results. This was followed by larger RCTs in ARDS, sepsis and the injured brain looking at mortality and other clinical endpoints. The 3 significant large RCTs investigated their role in the above ICU conditions all failed to show benefit.

The CRASH trial,[64] studied the role of steroids in all grades of traumatic brain injury. This was a large multinational trial with more than 10,000 patients, with India and the UK being among the largest contributors. They used a relatively high-dose of steroids. The loading dose was 2 g methylprednisolone (or placebo) over 1 h in a 100 mL infusion. The maintenance dose was 0.4 g methylprednisolone (or placebo) per h for 48 h in a 20 mL per h infusion. The investigators found that compared with placebo, the risk of death from all causes within 2 weeks was higher in the group allocated to receive corticosteroids (1052 [21.1%] vs. 893 [17.9%] deaths; relative risk 1.18 [95% CI 1.09–1.27]; $P = 0.0001$). The relative increase in deaths due to corticosteroids did not differ by injury severity ($P = 0{\cdot}22$) or time since injury ($P = 0.05$). A later analysis of the same data[65] found that the increase in mortality or in severe disability in the steroid treated patients persisted at 6 months. This increase was noted in all grades of severity of head injury. It is really difficult to justify any role for high-dose steroids in head injury after this study.

In earlier historical trials, high dose steroids in shock were associated with increased mortality, and steroids were abandoned for sepsis for many years. Later, there was a reemergence

Table 2. Historical studies of high does early steroids in ARDS and septic shock.

Study	Patients	Dose of MPS (methylprednisolone)	Results (MPS versus Placebo)
Bone 1987	304, sepsis	30 mg/kg x 4, within 2hrs of diagnosis of sepsis	Incidence of ARDS 32% vs. 25% Reversal 31% vs. 61%, *P*=0.004 14 day mortality 52% vs. 22%, *P*=0.004
Bernard 1987	99, ARDS	30 mg/kg 6 hourly for 24 hours	Mortality 60% vs. 63% Reversal of ARDS 36% vs. 39%
Luce J, 1988	87, septic shock	30 mg/kg 6 hourly for 24 hours	Progression to ARDS 34% vs. 38% Mortality 58% vs. 54%
Weigelt J, 1985	81 ventilated patients, high risk of ARDS	30 mg/kg 6 hourly for 48 hours	Developed ARDS 64% vs. 33% Infections 77% vs. 43%

High-dose steroids should definitely not be used in patients with head injury.

of lower dose steroids, not for their immune modulating effect, but as a "stress dose", apparently to sensitize catecholamine receptors. An earlier trial,[66] showed some benefit in "non responders". These were patients who mounted a subnormal response to an ACTH challenge, and the theory was that they could not produce as much steroid as they needed, and hence, would benefit from supplementation. The CORTICUS trial,[67] was conducted to resolve these issues. They studied about 500 patients using 50 mg 6 hourly of hydrocortisone for 5 days and then tapering over another 6 days. They concluded that hydrocortisone did not improve survival or reversal of shock among patients with septic shock, either overall or among patients who did not have a response to corticotropin, although hydrocortisone hastened reversal of shock among patients in whom shock was reversed. Some people have felt that the study was negative because they included moderately and severely ill patients while the earlier Annane trial only included severe sepsis. It is still not uncommon to see these stress dose steroids being used in sepsis despite the negative CORTICUS trials.

Steroids seem to be a good idea in ARDS, which is essentially an inflammatory condition of the lung. After the early historical studies showed harm, their use decreased. There was a resurgence for its use, later in ARDS to prevent delayed fibro-proliferation. This was based on a study of 24 patients by Meduri[68] where 2 mg/kg methylprednisolone was used for 2 weeks and then tapered for another 17 days. It was started late, after a week of ARDS. It showed some promise and prompted the ARDS-net group to conduct a definitive trial, called the Late Rescue Steroid trial (LaRS). The LaRS study[69] steroid regime was similar to the above Meduri trial for the first 2 weeks, but tapered off more rapidly over 10 days. They concluded that their results do not support the routine use of methylprednisolone for persistent ARDS despite the improvement in cardiopulmonary physiology. In addition, starting methylprednisolone therapy more than 2 weeks after the onset of ARDS may increase the risk of death. It is worth noting in this particular trial that there was a marked improvement seen in the early phase of steroid therapy, both in terms of pulmonary function and weaning off ventilator. But this was counterbalanced by a higher incidence of delayed deterioration and re-ventilation in the steroid group. This delayed deterioration was attributed to steroid induced neuromuscular weakness and not due to sepsis. Over a period of weeks, the initial gains were matched by the delayed complication, with no net benefit. Critics of this study felt the steroid regime was inappropriate. Another unsatisfactory aspect to this trial was a change of assumptions in the power calculation and sample size. (The initial power calculation stated that a minimum number of 400 patients were needed to have a statistical power of 85% to detect a 15% absolute reduction in mortality compared to an expected 50% in untreated patients. The revised power calculation stated that a minimum number of 180 patients were needed to have a statistical power of 85% to detect a 20% absolute reduction in mortality compared to an expected 40% in untreated patients. This was cleared by data and safety monitoring board). It is probably unrealistic to expect steroids to decrease the mortality from 40 to 20%, making one wonder if the negative result was due to lack of steroid effect or poor trial design.

Meduri then conducted another trial[70] with 91 patients using a smaller dose of steroids of 1 mg/kg for 2 weeks and then tapered over another 2 weeks. Another significant difference was that it was started early, in the first 3 days of ARDS. This has been labeled as a positive trial as there was greater benefit in the first week. However, other than ICU mortality, there was no mortality benefit at 7 days, 28 days, 60 day, 6 months and 1 year. Meduri concluded his paper with the following two sentences. "A larger trial is necessary to confirm the mortality findings of this study. In a future trial, we recommend adding stratification by shock at study entry, and strict implementation and monitoring of a ventilator and weaning protocol".

To summarize, high-dose steroids should definitely not be used in head injury and no specific regime of steroids in ARDS and sepsis have been shown to improve major clinical outcomes in large randomized trials.

The VOMIT Syndrome: Victim of Medical Imaging Technology

In 2002, Richard Hayward, a consultant neurosurgeon from Great Ormond Street Hospital for Children, London, introduced the above term in the medical literature, calling it an acronym of our times.[71] The "I" could equally be any medical Investigation, not limited to Imaging. He started with a couple of illustrative cases where an incidental finding provoked undue anxiety (cyst in the brain of a child with headache, and possible lumbar syrinx in a 15 year old with a low back pain). Most practising clinicians would have seen variations of this: An incidental finding followed by internet research by the concerned patient and family. Our only job in

In ARDS and sepsis, no specific regime of steroids has been shown to improve major clinical outcomes in large randomized trials.

An ethical part of our contemporary role as physicians is to prevent our patients from becoming victims of medical imaging technology.

this situation is to offer reassurance. But many of us would also have seen unnecessary treatment or surgery by either well meaning doctors or by unscrupulous doctors, with no real clinical benefit for the health or symptomatic relief of the patient. The author goes on to state that imaging centres as a business are now a reality, and many patients will self-refer themselves to these obliging centres, and we doctors have to adapt to this new reality. An ethical part of our contemporary job plan is to prevent our patients from becoming victims of medical imaging technology.

A decade later, we are still no closer to solving this problem which is widespread and epidemic.[72] We highlight one study to demonstrate that routine scanning may have consequences worse than undue anxiety and unnecessary treatment and procedures.[73] The authors sought to analyze whether the use of abdominal CT among patients with abdominal injury requiring laparotomy results in a significant delay and a higher risk of poor outcome. They did a retrospective analysis of trauma patients with SBP < 90 needing urgent laparotomy (< 90 min of arrival). They analysed 3,218 such patients with logistic regression and found that doing an abdominal CT was independently associated with more than a 70% higher risk of mortality (odds ratios, 1.71; 95% CI, 1.2–2.2; *P*= 0.001). They concluded that a delay secondary to abdominal imaging among patients who require operative intervention results in an independent higher risk of mortality.

Conclusions

The list of routine yet unproven therapies used in ICU appears endless. The previous 3 chapters have looked at the evidence behind many of our standard therapies and the majority have failed to demonstrate patient benefit. Many have shown harm. In this context, it appears intuitive to be restrictive rather than liberal when selecting therapies for the critically ill in ICU. This is not a lazy approach; rather it is a well-researched and carefully thought out strategy. As an additional benefit, being restrictive will also prevent waste of resources, and in today's world, this equally applies to the rich and poor parts of the world.

This may also appear to be a defeatist or a nihilistic approach, but that is far from true. We clearly believe that our major default therapies such as mechanical ventilation, vasoactive medication and renal replacement therapy are lifesaving. But we also feel that every therapy we routinely use needs study, and needs to show patient benefit. We only state that blind belief, based on some personal experience is not good enough. This quote from 170 years ago summarizes our position.

Of those who recover from a state approaching to dissolution a greater number will owe their recovery to unassisted nature than to the most judicious treatment. But let us not on this account undervalue the knowledge which physiological investigations throw on this interesting subject.

– Sir Benjamin Brodie, 1846

References

1. A Malhotra, D Maughan, J Ansell, *et al.* Choosing Wisely in the UK: the Academy of Medical Royal Colleges' initiative to reduce the harms of too much medicine. *BMJ* 2015;350:h2308.
2. Atul Gawande. Overkill. An avalanche of unnecessary medical care is harming patients physically and financially. What can we do about it? *Annals of Health Care* May 11, 2015.
3. The New Yoker and Atul Gawande. The Cost Conundrum.
4. Goldacre. Bad Science 2009:pp83 Harper Collins.
5. Shang A, Huwiler-Müntener K, Nartey L,*et al.* Are the clinical effects of homoeopathy placebo effects? Comparative study of placebo-controlled trials of homoeopathy and allopathy. *Lancet* 2005;366:726–32.
6. Takala. Increased mortality associated with growth hormone treatment in critically ill adults. *N Engl J Med* 1999;341:785–92.
7. Jennifer S, Temel MD, Joseph A, *et al.* Early palliative care for patients with metastatic non–small-cell lung cancer. *N Engl J Med* 2010;363:733–42.
8. Jena AB, Prasad V, Goldman DP, *et al.* Mortality and treatment patterns among patients hospitalized with acute cardiovascular conditions during dates of national cardiology meetings. *JAMA Intern Med* 2015;175(2):237–44.
9. Cornet AD, Kooter AJ, Peters MJ, *et al.* Supplemental oxygen therapy in medical emergencies: more harm than benefit? *Arch Intern Med* 2012;172(3):289–90. www.archinternmed.com
10. Kilgannon JH, Jones AE, Shapiro NI, *et al.* Association between arterial hyperoxia following resuscitation from cardiac arrest and in-hospital mortality. *JAMA* 2010;303(21):2165–71.
11. Austin MA, Wills E, Blizzard L, *et al.* High flow oxygen increases mortality in chronic obstructive pulmonary disease patients in a pre-hospital setting: a randomized trial. *BMJ* 2010;341:c5462.
12. Stub D, Smith K, Bernard S, *et al.* Air versus oxygen in st-segment elevation myocardial infarction. *Circulation* 2015;131(24):2143–50.
13. Van Hoeyweghen RJ, Bossaert LL, Mullie A, *et al.* Quality and efficiency of bystander CPR. *Resuscitation* 1993;26:47–52.
14. Hallstrom A, Cobb L, Johnson E, *et al.* Cardiopulmonary resuscitation by chest compression alone or with mouth-to-mouth ventilation. *N Engl J Med* 2000;342:1546–53.
15. Page RL, Joglar JA, Kowal RC, *et al.* Use of automated external defibrillators by a U.S. airline. *N Engl J Med* 2000;343:1210–16.

16. Valenzuela TD, Roe DJ, Nichol G, *et al.* Outcomes of rapid defibrillation by security officers after cardiac arrest in casinos. *N Engl J Med* 2000;343:1206–9.
17. Chan PS, Krumholz HM, Spertus JA, *et al.* Automated external defibrillators and survival after in-hospital cardiac arrest. *JAMA* 2010;304:2129–36.
18. Hasegawa K, Hiraide A, Chang Y, *et al.* Association of prehospital advanced airway management with neurologic outcome and survival in patients with out-of hospital cardiac arrest. *JAMA* 2013;309:257–66.
19. Pearson JW, Redding JS.. The role of epinephrine in cardiac resuscitation. *Anesthesia and Analgesia* 1963;42:599–606
20. Stiell IG, Hebert PC, Weitzman BN, *et al.* High-dose epinephrine in adult cardiac arrest. *N Engl J Med* 1992;327:1045–50.
21. Brown CG, Martin DR, Pepe PE, *et al.* A comparison of standard-dose and high-dose epinephrine in cardiac arrest outside the hospital. *N Engl J Med* 1992;327:1051–55.
22. Gueugniaud PY, Mols P, Goldstein P, *et al.* A comparison of repeated high doses and repeated standard doses of epinephrine for cardiac arrest outside the hospital. *N Engl J Med* 1998;339:1595–601.
23. Jacobs IG, Finn JC, Jelinek GA, *et al.* Effect of adrenaline on survival in out-of-hospital cardiac arrest: A randomized double-blind placebo-controlled trial. *Resuscitation* 2011;82:1138–43.
24. Soar J, Nolan JP.. Adrenaline-Proven benefit in cardiac arrest at last?" *Resuscitation* 2011;82:1115–16.
25. Olasveengen TM, Sunde K, Brunborg C, *et al.* Intravenous drug administration during out-of-hospital cardiac arrest: a randomized trial. *JAMA* 2009;302:2222–29.
26. Olasveengen T, Wik L, Sunde K, *et al.* Outcome when adrenaline (epinephrine) was actually given vs. not given - post hoc analysis of a randomized clinical trial. *Resuscitation* 2012;83:327–32.
27. Hagihara A, Hasegawa M, Abe T, *et al.* Prehospital epinephrine use and survival among patients with out-of-hospital cardiac arrest. *JAMA* 2012;307:1161–68.
28. Nakahara S, Tomio J, Takahashi H, *et al.* Evaluation of pre-hospital administration of adrenaline (epinephrine) by emergency medical services for patients with out of hospital cardiac arrest in Japan: controlled propensity matched retrospective cohort study. *BMJ* 2013;347:f6829.
29. Dumas F, Bougouin W, Geri G, *et al.* Is epinephrine during cardiac arrest associated with worse outcomes in resuscitated patients? *J Am Coll Cardiol* 2014;64:2360–67.
30. Lin S, Callaway C W, Shah PS, *et al.* Adrenaline for out-of-hospital cardiac arrest resuscitation: A systematic review and meta-analysis of randomized controlled trials. *Resuscitation* 2014;85:732–40.
31. Patanwala AE, Slack MK, Martin JR, *et al.* Effect of epinephrine on survival after cardiac arrest: a systematic review and meta-analysis. *Minerva Anestesiol* 2014;80:831–43.
32. The Hypothermia after Cardiac Arrest Study Group. Mild therapeutic hypothermia to improve the neurologic outcome after cardiac arrest. *N Engl J Med* 2002;346:549–56.
33. Bernard SA, Gray TW, Buist MD, *et al.* Treatment of comatose survivors of out-of- hospital cardiac arrest with induced hypothermia. *N Engl J Med* 2002;346:557–63
34. Nielsen N, Wetterslev J, Cronberg T, *et al.* Targeted temperature management at 33 degree C versus 36 degree C after cardiac arrest. *N Engl J Med* 2013;369:2197–206.
35. Moler FW, Silverstein FS, Holubkov R, *et al.* Therapeutic hypothermia after out-of-hospital cardiac arrest in children. *N Engl J Med* 2015;372(20):1898–908.
36. Hébert PC, Wells G, Blajchman MA, *et al.* A multicenter, randomized, controlled clinical trial of transfusion requirements in critical care. Transfusion Requirements in Critical Care Investigators, Canadian Critical Care Trials Group.*NEJM* 1999;340:409–17.
37. Wu WC, Rathore SS, Wang Y, *et al.* Blood transfusion in elderly patients with acute myocardial infarction. *N Engl J Med* 2001;345:1230–36.
38. Hébert PC, Yetisir E, Martin C, *et al.* Is a low transfusion threshold safe in critically ill patients with cardiovascular diseases? *Crit Care Med* 2001;29:227–34.

39. Vincent JL, Sakr Y, Sprung C, *et al.* Are blood transfusions associated with greater mortality rates? Results of the sepsis occurrence in acutely ill patients study. *Anesthesiology* 2008;108:31–9.
40. Park DW, Chun BC, Kwon SS, *et al.* Red blood cell transfusions are associated with lower mortality in patients with severe sepsis and septic shock: a propensity matched analysis. *Crit Care Med* 2012;40: 3140–45.
41. Holst LB, Haase N, Wetterslev J, *et al.*Lower versus higher hemoglobin threshold for transfusion in septic shock. *N Engl J Med* 2014;371:1381–91.
42. Lacroix J, Hébert PC, Fergusson DA, *et al.* Age of Transfused Blood in Critically Ill Adults. *N Engl J Med* 2015;372:1410–8.
43. ESICM Systematic Review Group. Clinical Evidence in Intensive Care-2011 Nutrition and Metabolism. Section 10: pp208–212. Medizinisch Wissenschaftliche Verlagsgesellschaft
44. Harvey SE, Parrott F, Harrison DA, *et al.* Trial of the route of early nutritional support in critically ill adults. *N Engl J Med* 2014;371:1673–84.
45. Casaer MP, Mesotten D, Hermans G, *et al.* Early versus late parenteral nutrition in critically ill adults. *N Engl J Med* 2011;365:506–17.
46. Casaer M, Wilmer A, Hermans G, *et al.* Role of disease and macronutrient dose in the randomized controlled EPaNIC trial: a post hoc analysis. *Am J Respir Crit Care Med* 2013;187:247–55.
47. Doig GS, Simpson F, Sweetman EA, *et al.* Early parenteral nutrition in critically ill patients with short-term relative contraindications to early enteral nutrition: a randomized controlled trial. *JAMA* 2013;309(20): 2130–38.
48. Heys SD, Walker LG, Smith I, *et al.* Enteral nutritional supplementation with key nutrients in patients with critical illness and cancer: a meta-analysis of randomized controlled clinical trials. *Ann Surg* 1999;229: 467–77.
49. Beale RJ, Bryg DJ, Bihari DJ. Immunonutrition in the critically ill: a systematic review of clinical outcome. *Crit Care Med* 1999;27:2799–2805.
50. Galbán C, Montejo JC, Mesejo A, *et al.* An immune-enhancing enteral diet reduces mortality rate and episodes of bacteremia in septic intensive care unit patients. *Crit Care Med* 2000;28:643–48.
51. Canadian Clinical Practice Guidelines www.criticalcarenutrition.com March 2013r
52. Heyland D, Muscedere J, Wischmeyer PE, *et al.* A randomized trial of glutamine and antioxidants in critically ill patients. *N Engl J Med* 2013;368:1489–97.
53. Furnary AP, Zerr KJ, Grunkemeier GL, *et al.* Continuous intravenous insulin infusion reduces the incidence of deep sternal wound infection in diabetic patients after cardiac surgical procedures. *Ann Thorac Surg* 1999;67:352–62.
54. Furnary AP, Gao G, Grunkemeier GL, *et al.* Continuous insulin infusion reduces mortality in patients with diabetes undergoing coronary artery bypass grafting. *Journal of Thoracic and Cardiovascular Surgery* 2003;125 (5):1007–19
55. van den Berghe G, Wouters P, Weekers F, *et al.* Intensive insulin therapy in critically ill patients. *N Engl J Med* 2001;345:1359–67.
56. Van den Berghe G, Wilmer A, Hermans G, *et al.* Intensive insulin therapy in the medical ICU. *N Engl J Med* 2006;354:449–61.
57. Brunkhorst FM, Kuhnt E, Engel C, *et al.* Intensive insulin in patients with severe sepsis and septic shock is associated with an increased rate of hypoglycemia – results from a randomized multicenter study (VISEP). *Infection* 2005;33:19–20
58. Preiser JC, Devos P, *et al.* A prospective randomised multi-centre controlled trial on tight glucose control by intensive insulin therapy in adult intensive care units: the Glucontrol study. *Intensive Care Med* 2009;35(10):1738–48.

59. NICE-SUGAR Study Investigators, Finfer S, Chittock DR, *et al.* Intensive versus Conventional Glucose Control in Critically Ill Patients. *N Engl J Med* 2009;360(13):1283–97.

60. Guyatt GH, Akl EA, Crowther M, *et al.* Antithrombotic Therapy and Prevention of Thrombosis, 9th ed: American College of Chest Physicians Evidence-Based Clinical Practice Guidelines. *Chest.* 2012;141(2_ suppl):7S–47S

61. Kakkar AK, Cimminiello C, Goldhaber SZ, *et al.* Low-molecular-weight heparin and mortality in acutely ill medical patients. *N Engl J Med* 2011;365:2463–72.

62. The PROTECT Investigators for the Canadian Critical Care Trials Group and the Australian and New Zealand Intensive Care Society Clinical Trials Group. Dalteparin versus unfractionated heparin in critically ill patients. *N Engl J Med* 2011;364:1305–14.

63. Sharrock NE, Gonzalez Della Valle A, Go G, *et al* Potent anticoagulants are associated with a higher all-cause mortality rate after hip and knee arthroplasty. *Clin Orthop Relat Res* 2008;466:714–21.

64. Roberts I, Yates D, Sandercock P, *et al.* Effect of intravenous corticosteroids on death within 14 days in 10 008 adults with clinically significant head injury (MRC CRASH trial): randomized placebo-controlled trial. *Lancet* 2004;364:1321–28.

65. Edwards P, Arango M, Balica L, *et al.* Final results of MRC CRASH, a randomized placebo-controlled trial of intravenous corticosteroid in adults with head injury-outcomes at 6 months. *Lancet* 2005;365:1957–59.

66. Annane D, S.bille V, Charpentier C, *et al.* Effect of treatment with low doses of hydrocortisone and fludrocortisone on mortality in patients with septic shock. *JAMA* 2002;288:862–71.

67. Sprung CL, Annane D, Keh D, *et al.* Hydrocortisone therapy for patients with septic shock. *N Engl J Med* 2008;358:111–24.

68. Meduri GU, Headley AS, Golden E, *et al.* Effect of prolonged methylprednisolone therapy in unresolving acute respiratory distress syndrome: a randomized controlled trial. *JAMA* 1998;280(2):159–65.

69. Steinberg KP, Hudson LD, Goodman RB, *et al.* Efficacy and safety of corticosteroids for persistent acute respiratory distress syndrome. *N Engl J Med* 2006;354:1671–84.

70. Meduri GU, Golden E, Freire AX, *et al.* Methylprednisolone infusion in early severe ARDS: results of a randomized controlled trial. *CHEST* 2007;131:954–63.

71. Richard Hayward VOMIT (victims of modern imaging technology)—an acronym for our times. *BMJ* 2003;326:1273.

72. Hillman BJ, Goldsmith JC. The uncritical use of high-tech medical imaging. *N Engl J Med* 2010;363(1):4-6.

73. Neal MD, Peitzman AB, Forsythe RM, *et al.* Over reliance on computed tomography imaging in patients with severe abdominal injury: is the delay worth the risk? *J Trauma* 2011;70:278–84.

Pitfalls 6-8

The patient has stabilized and is showing signs of recovery. The inotropes are off and the patient is awake and alert on Pressure Support Ventilation (PSV). That day, there is a staff shortage. Additionally, a few have left the ICU in response to a cardiopulmonary resuscitation (CPR) code which turns out to be a mock CPR analysis by the inspectors of the national accreditation board for hospitals (NABH). (The ICU team had stated that such a mock drill is unnecessary as the yearly CPR and RRT [Rapid Response Team] statistics were available for the NABH, but the hospital administrators overrode them). There was no nurse in the patients' cubicle and the patient self extubated. The patient rapidly worsens, and the resident is not in the ICU. The RRT-CPR team is paged. The patient is manually ventilated with face mask and bag till the ICU resident returns from the mock drill. During the intubation attempt, the laryngoscope light stops working and it takes time to find another one. The suction too gives trouble, further delaying the intubation. The patient is reintubated, but it is a difficult one done after multiple attempts. There is desaturation and severe bradycardia requiring a short period of CPR. After intubation, the patient rapidly stabilizes but remains unresponsive neurologically during initial assessment after muscle relaxant has worn off. The ICU resident is then requested to return briefly for the mock drill but asks a colleague to cover till he returns or till the next shift resident takes over care of the ICU. The ICU consultant is then informed about the event. On the evening round, the relatives inform the primary admitting consultant that there was some problem, but they are not clear what happened. The primary consultant is unable to find any notes documenting the event. He notes the oxygen saturation is 92% and the patient is still unresponsive and orders 100% oxygen to be given, as per his specialty guidelines, to help the brain recover. A neurologist requests a magnetic resonance imaging (MRI) followed by an electroencephalography (EEG), as per his specialty guidelines. The patient recovers consciousness and is fully lucid in the next 6-12 hours, but the MRI and EEG are still done later as the neurologist and primary consultant feel it would be safer. Monitoring in the MRI is limited to pulse oximetry and when the patient is moved out, he is found to be hypotensive. A fluid bolus does not reverse the hypotension and noradrenaline is restarted. The blood pressure (BP) slowly increases but the patient remains oliguric and the next day's renal parameters are worse. He then stabilizes over the next 48-72 hours, the inotropes are withdrawn and the renal parameters become normal.

What are the Pitfalls?

Pitfalls 6-8

Inadequate ICU Infrastructure

There are several pitfalls in this scenario.

First, safety protocols for emergency intubation were not followed, as one usually checks the light of the laryngoscope, keeps a spare one ready and checks the suction before the first attempt at intubation. Second, there was blind and inappropriate adherence to some guidelines regarding 100% oxygen and the need for imaging and EEG following a short witnessed cardiac arrest.

Next, there was poor communication and documentation at every step of the way. The resident should have been alerted to the possibility of a difficult intubation, as this happened at the initial intubation and should have requested consultant backup. Once the situation had been reversed, all the appropriate consultants and the family should have been informed as to the incident, and this should also have been documented in detail.

Lastly, there was a failure of adequate staffing, and in this scenario, further removing ICU staff for a mock CPR as part of an accreditation process significantly decreased safety standards.

Additionally, it reflects a complete failure on the part of the accreditation committee to understand the nature of quality assessment. Quality is usually assessed on outcomes. If outcome data is not available, then compliance with set standards is a surrogate for quality. But in this case, despite there being outcome data, the ritual of evaluating compliance was carried out.

In the introduction, it was stated that the intensivist has two roles. First to identify and reverse the triggering illness, and secondly, to keep the patient alive till the illness has been reversed. There is actually a third role. And that is to ensure the ICU has an adequate infrastructure to deliver the above two roles. Part of this infrastructure is a set of pragmatic safety protocols, a clear system to ensure communication between all ICU and other medical personnel and relatives, a disciplined system of documentation, and also to ensure an adequate number of trained staff are present in the ICU.

Pitfall No. 6

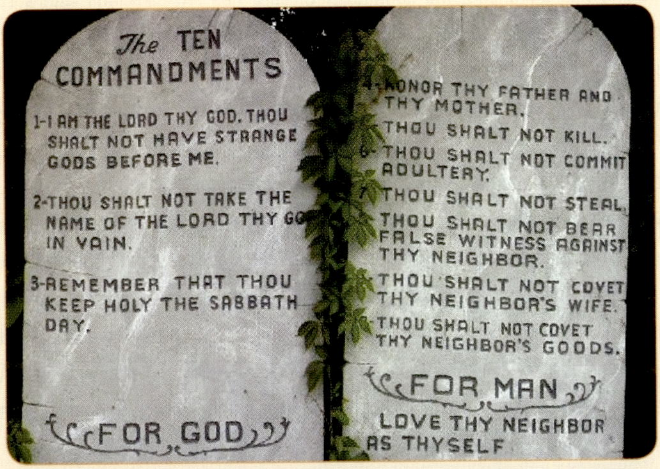

The TEN COMMANDMENTS
1-I AM THE LORD THY GOD. THOU SHALT NOT HAVE STRANGE GODS BEFORE ME.
2-THOU SHALT NOT TAKE THE NAME OF THE LORD THY GO
IN VAIN.
3-REMEMBER THAT THOU KEEP HOLY THE SABBATH DAY.
FOR GOD
HONOR THY FATHER AND THY MOTHER.
THOU SHALT NOT KILL.
6-THOU SHALT NOT COMMIT ADULTERY.
THOU SHALT NOT STEAL.
THOU SHALT NOT BEAR FALSE WITNESS AGAINST THY NEIGHBOR.
THOU SHALT NOT COVET THY NEIGHBOR'S WIFE.
THOU SHALT NOT COVET THY NEIGHBOR'S GOODS.
FOR MAN
LOVE THY NEIGHBOR AS THYSELF

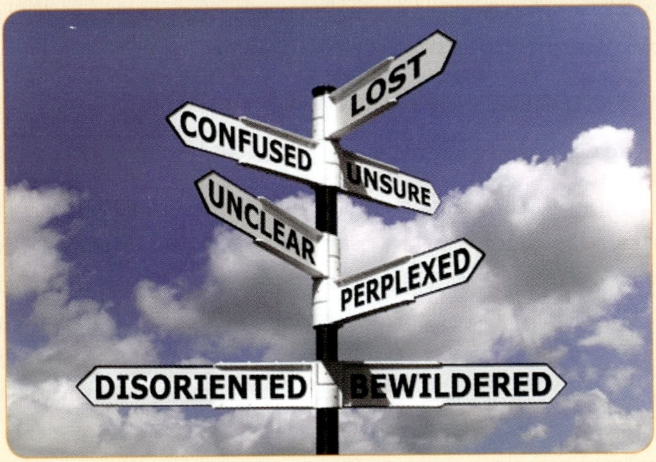

LOST
CONFUSED
UNSURE
UNCLEAR
PERPLEXED
DISORIENTED
BEWILDERED

Pitfall No. 6

Failure to Appropriately Use Protocols and Guidelines

As medicine has advanced, the complexity of care has left clinicians with a staggering amount of literature with some very conflicting evidence. Busy clinical lives make filtering through and keeping up to date with the latest evidence a practical nightmare. Guidelines were initially developed as an aid to assist clinicians with their decision making and in some ways to streamline and standardise the care provided and thus improve efficiency and patient safety. Over the years there has been a proliferation of guidelines for anything and everything possible. As an example, the Agency for Healthcare Research and Quality's National Guideline Clearing house in the US, currently contains nearly 2350 guidelines under the heading of "diseases" alone and a total of 100 guidelines in progress. National Institute of Clinical Excellence (NICE) in the UK, currently has 229 published guidelines and another 376 in development. Of the published guidelines 158 are clinical guidelines. The Guidelines International Network, on the other hand, has 6470 guidelines from 96 organizations from 83 countries... A mindboggling array of guidelines!

Along with these nationally and internationally available guidelines, there are local protocols and policies that clinicians are expected to be aware of and follow.

Where then does this leave the practicing clinician?

Firstly, the definitions of the terms guidelines, protocols and policies can be confusing.

By definition a "clinical practice guideline" is an evidence based recommendation for clinicians about specific conditions and their management, whereas a "protocol" is an agreed rigid framework that precisely details the how, when, where and what care is provided. A "policy" on the other hand, is a contractually binding, formally written statement, of a specific action that needs to be taken in a specific situation. Protocols and policies are based on

Some deride protocols as cook book medicine, to be followed by those incapable of independent thought, while others proclaim that failure to follow guidelines is akin to negligence.

the clinical practice guideline. Therefore, how good a protocol or policy is depends on how strong the evidence in the guideline is.

Historically one of the first policies was created in 1938 by the American Academy of Pediatrics followed in 1959 by problem specific advisories from the American College of Obstetrics and Gynecology.[1] But it was in 1986, when the American Society of Anesthesiologists (ASA) 12 point standards for basic anesthetic monitoring, was published which not only improved patient care but also appeared to have reduced malpractice losses in the US and thus brought about a reduction in insurance premiums, that gave guidelines the prominence they appear to enjoy today.[2,3]

Protocols are designed to prevent disasters; They are not designed to promote excellence.

– William Shoemaker

This line summarizes the current schizophrenic approach of the medical community to protocols and guidelines. Some deride protocols as cook book medicine, to be followed by those incapable of independent thought, while others proclaim that failure to follow guidelines is akin to negligence. The latter seem to be gaining ground and there are a large number of physicians who now defensively follow protocols they do not think effective.

A suggested pragmatic approach, or dare we say it, an evidence-free guideline for following guidelines, could be

- Obsessively follow pragmatic protocols to enhance safety
- Largely follow other guidelines based on high quality evidence
- Resist slavishly following other guidelines based on poor quality evidence.

Two analogies from sports are worth considering. To win a race, a Formula 1 car first needs to be reliable enough to last the distance. This will get it to the finish line, but will not ensure a win. The car also needs to have a high performance and the driver needs to be able to utilize that performance to its maximum. But high performance and skillful driving alone too will not be enough, as breaking down in the lead position earns 0 points for driver and team. Similarly, a football team needs to have both, a tight defense and a creative and effective offence. Matches and leagues can only be won when both are functioning optimally. In ICU, to maximize good clinical outcomes, ICUs need to have tight protocols on basic safety, but to have sound but flexible approaches to other aspects of therapy.

Preventing Disasters

The data from the World Health Organization (WHO) Patient Safety programme, launched in 2004, suggests that in the developed world nearly 1 in 10 patients suffer a healthcare related adverse event. The number is probably higher in the developing world as the data available is patchy although a study published by the Harvard School of Public Health estimated that of every 100 hospitalizations, there were approximately 14.2 adverse events in high income countries and 12.7 in low and medium income countries.[4] The 1999 Institute of medicine report "To err is Human: Building a safer Health System" suggested that between 44,000 – 98,000 Americans die every year as a result of medical errors taking the estimated cost of preventable adverse events to anything between $17 - $29 billion. The current estimate is pegged even higher at approximately 210,000 – 400,000 deaths per year.[5] Medical errors ranked third as the leading cause of death in the US in 2010.[6] Another unpalatable truth of clinical care and medical errors is litigation. In the NHS clinical negligence claims rose by 17.9% from 2012/2013 to 2013/2014.

All this points to a need for safer systems in healthcare, if we are to reduce preventable adverse events. Guidelines and protocols form the backbone of present day patient safety initiatives. Although, guidelines allow for leeway thus helping provide individualised care, protocols, by their very nature, are rigid and deviation from established protocols is frowned upon. It's impossible to have a protocol in place for every eventuality on intensive care, but protocols for simple everyday activities such as venous thromboembolism (VTE) prophylaxis, infection control, stress ulcer prevention help standardise care and reduce adverse events.

One initiative that has improved patient safety with regards to surgical interventions is the WHO Surgical Safety Checklist, a 19 item tool, designed to improve communication and consistency of care to reduce complications associated with surgery. The 2009 NEJM

Guidelines promoting basic safety should be obsessively followed.

Checklists can improve outcomes.

publication highlighted a reduction in in-house mortality to 0.8% from 1.5% following the introduction of the checklist and a drop in complications from 11 to 7%.[7] In a small surgical study published in 2009 looking at surgical adverse events in tertiary hospitals in Delhi, India, 31.5% preventable adverse events (PAE) were identified. Of these 84.3% were system errors which included a lack of protocols and policies e.g. management of infection control post operatively, and 82.7% operative errors which included wrong choice of surgery.[8] In situations like this implementation of practical infection control protocols and a surgical checklist would help reduce PAEs.

As critical care gets more complex inconsistencies in decision making, whether due to case mix or the availability of resources and facilities crop up. Care bundles, a group of evidence based interventions, were introduced based on the assumption that there would be an improvement in patient safety, if the interventions were implemented together versus if they were implemented independently. On ICU the most commonly used bundles are the ventilator care bundle and the central line bundle. The Michigan keystone project in 2006 which was implemented across 103 hospitals showed a drop in catheter related infections per 1000 catheter days from 2.7 to 0 in 3 months following the implementation of the central line care bundle.[9] Care bundles were also introduced as part of the Surviving Sepsis Campaign. One of the guiding principles of implementation of these care bundles is 100% compliance. Achieving 100% compliance requires all stakeholders on intensive care especially the medical and nursing teams, to accept and participate in the implementation of the care bundles. These care bundles have also evolved over time with their components being adapted/discarded based on new evidence.

The human factor aspect that contributes to medical errors still remains and cannot be completely eliminated. The only way for an individual to reduce the risk of causing inadvertent harm is by being "obsessive" about patient safety. For this obsession with patient safety to work requires buy in from all those working as part of a team. This includes developing unit protocols with the use of high quality, evidence backed guidelines as starters and then ensuring that the agreed protocols receive 100% compliance. But one must remember at all times that it's a patient that is being treated not a machine.

It is thus obvious that one should obsessively follow pragmatic protocols to enhance safety. There is also no disadvantage in checking the function of the laryngoscope and suction prior to an elective intubation. There is also no down side to have a spare laryngoscope and endotracheal tube before an elective intubation. Similarly, adequate venous access, adequate monitoring and staff to assist are all necessary safety components to ensure a smooth intubation. This kind of obsession for all major ICU procedures such as vascular cannulation and tracheostomy, or when setting up a mechanical ventilator or a hemofilter, go a long way in preventing avoidable complications. There is a clear agreement and supporting data to suggest that this kind of obsessive use of safety protocols should be the standard of care, and failure to follow these would be considered as negligent.

Limitations of Clinical Guidelines

Users of clinical guidelines should be aware of their many limitations. We briefly cover some of them.

Clinical studies rely on probability, and the whole aim of a study is to evaluate if the response seen could be random, or due to the therapeutic intervention. This requires clinicians to evaluate the degree of certainty of the therapy being effective, and apply it to an individual clinical situation. Unfortunately, a guideline does not convey this uncertainty, and a useful suggestion gets translated into a black and white recommendation. Some guidelines use the terms "we recommend" or "we suggest" to convey this, but for most readers, it becomes difficult to ignore the recommendation.

Many guidelines are based on studies with small numbers. It is highly probable, that many will have to be reviewed when larger studies are done, but again, the clinician interprets the recommendation as something that must be done. Similarly, many guidelines are based on studies with only surrogate endpoints. Once they become a recommendation, clinicians often assume it actually helps patients by improving clinical outcomes. Worse, many guidelines are based on post hoc subgroup analysis. These are actually hypotheses worth studying, but once they are framed as a recommendation, clinicians assume that they have been adequately studied and proven.

Users of clinical guidelines should be aware of their many limitations. Clinicians must evaluate the degree of certainty of the therapy being effective, and apply it to an individual clinical situation.

Too many guidelines, too little clarity.

There have been reviews on how to create guidelines,[10] and amazingly, in a random sample of 130 guidelines, less than 30-50% of guidelines actually follow guidelines on how to frame their own guidelines.[11]

A potentially worrying trend is the financial support of industry in the creation of guidelines.[12-14] Statements are made about independence of the panelists, but conflicts of interest are a fact of life. In the above survey <50% gave information regarding Conflicts Of Interest (COI). When supplied, financial or intellectual COI were the norm, with 71.4% of committee chairpersons and 90.5% of co-chairpersons declaring such a COI. The review also noted that differences of opinion were rarely described and the benefits of recommendations were enumerated more often than potential harms.[15]

Majority of panelists on controversial new cholesterol guideline have current or recent ties to drug manufacturers.[16]

Yet another worry about guidelines is that compliance with guidelines is viewed as a sign of high quality medicine. This is a very inadequate way of looking at quality. High quality medicine is based on good patient outcomes. Occasionally, it is difficult to measure these outcomes. In these circumstances it is justifiable to assume that if one adheres to the guideline, then clinical outcomes will automatically improve. To give a couple of examples: One can judge the CPR service of a hospital by reviewing their outcome data (hospital discharge with good neurological function) or one could stage a mock code and record how well the drill scored against the guidelines. Obviously, if one knows the outcome data is significantly better than average reported in the literature, one would presume it was a good CPR service, regardless of the score in a mock drill. Similarly, one could capture data as to how frequently ICU personnel washed their hands in the ICU and grade the infection control on the percentage of compliance. But, the actual rates of ICU acquired infections would serve as a much better marker of the quality of the infection control practices in that ICU.

Most worrying is that guidelines have been demonstrated to cause harm, sometimes extensive harm. We cite three examples.

In the 1990s, steroids in spinal trauma were considered a "Standard of Care". In March 2013, the Congress of Neurological Surgeons reversed this guideline and stated that there was no

Class I or Class II evidence supporting the benefit but there was Class I, II, and III evidence of harm including death.[17] In a poll of over 1000 neurosurgeons 11% believed the treatment was safe and effective and only 6% thought it should be a standard of care. Yet 60% said that they would prescribe the treatment and cited a fear of malpractice as the main reason to do so. So, a large number of patients got a potentially harmful treatment because it was recommended in a guideline.

An observational study looked at the impact of following antibiotic guidelines in an ICU for suspected resistant infections.[18] There was 34% mortality in the patients in whom the antibiotics complied with the guidelines and a lower mortality of 20% in those in whom the antibiotics did not comply with the guidelines. One should not read too much into this observational data, but at least it should raise questions about whether guidelines actually improve clinical outcomes.

The most worrying data that guidelines can cause widespread harm comes from a meta-analysis of introduction of β blockers peri-operatively among patients with ischemic heart disease (IHD).[19] The role of β blockers is to decrease the incidence of IHD events. And the drugs did achieve that. But despite a lower cardiovascular mortality, the treatment group had an increase in all cause mortality secondary to bradycardia, hypotension and stroke. The authors claimed that *"Refraining from this ESC guideline would therefore be expected to prevent up to 10,000 iatrogenic deaths each year in the UK."* If the last statistic is to be believed, one must accept that blind adherence to guidelines has the ability to cause patient harm on a massive scale.

These concerns about guidelines are being increasingly expressed in the medical literature.[20-25]

Guidelines for Clinical Therapy

An idealistic way of looking at guidelines is as follows. Clinicians best serve the patient by being updated. Guidelines set a common standard and are based on systematic reviews, rather than on expert opinion. Most clinicians do not have statistical and methodological skills to actually evaluate the vast data, so they should let appropriate clinical and academic

---

Refraining from the peri-operative beta blocker ESC guideline would be expected to prevent up to 10,000 iatrogenic deaths each year in the UK.

---

experts do the job. If clinicians have any doubts about the recommendations they explore the references.

Pragmatic approach to using guidelines

Considering all the above limitations of guidelines, it is clearly inappropriate to blindly follow all guidelines. The most pragmatic way to follow guidelines is to largely follow guidelines based on high quality evidence. In this context, this means large RCTs with clinically relevant outcomes. Guidelines based on low quality evidence or only on expert evidence should not be slavishly followed. Clinical judgment must dictate appropriate therapy, even if that means largely ignoring the guidelines. One hopes that in future, guidelines will transparently say that given the low level of evidence, the experts feel unable to give a recommendation.

Conclusion

A threefold approach to protocols and guidelines will help both, to prevent disasters and to promote excellence.

1. Obsessively follow pragmatic protocols to enhance safety
2. Largely follow other guidelines based on high quality evidence
3. Resist slavishly following other guidelines based on poor quality evidence

References

1. Napoli AM, Jagoda A. Clinical policies: Their history, future, medical legal implications, and growing importance to physicians. *J Emerg Med* 2007;33:425–32.
2. Eichorn J. Prevention of intraoperative anesthesia accidents and related severe injury through safety monitoring. *Anesthesiology* 1989;70:572–7.
3. Holzer J. The advent of clinical standards for professional liability. *QRB Qual Rev.Bull* 1990;16:71–9.
4. Jha AK, Larizgoitia I, Audera-Lopez C, *et al.* The global burden of unsafe medical care: analytic modelling of observational studies. *BMJ Qual Saf* 2013;22:809–15.
5. James JT. A new, evidence-based estimate of patient harms associated with hospital care. *J Patient Saf* 2013;9(3):122-8.
6. Heron M. Deaths: Leading causes for 2010. National Vital Statistics Report 2013; Vol 62 No. 6
7. Haynes AB, Weiser TG, Berry WR, *et al.* A surgical safety checklist to reduce morbidity and mortality in a global population. *N Engl J Med* 2009;360(5):491–99.
8. Kumar S, Chaudhary S. Medical errors and consequent adverse events in critically ill surgical patients in a tertiary care teaching hospital in Delhi. *J Emerg Trauma Shock* 2009;2(2):80–84.
9. Pronovost PJ, Goeschel CA, Colantuoni E, *et al.* Sustaining reductions in catheter related bloodstream infections in Michigan intensive care units: observational study. *Br Med J* 2010;340:c309.
10. Clinical Practice Guidelines We Can Trust www.iom.edu/cpgstandards March 2011

11. Kung J, Miller RR, Mackowiak PA. Failure of clinical practice guidelines to meet institute of medicine standards two more decades of little, if any, progress. *Arch Intern Med.* 2012;172:1628–33.
12. Goldacre B, Carroll D, Hall E. Guidelines for collaboration with industry should be transparent. *BMJ* 2013;347:f6100.
13. Torjesen I. Three quarters of guideline panellists have ties to the drug industry. *BMJ* 2013;347:f4998.
14. Barraclough K. Beware the influence of the "SIF" (single issue fanatic) in clinical guidelines. *BMJ* 2013;347:f4719.
15. Peter J Gordon, Sian F Gordon. SIGN should be transparent about competing interests in all current guidelines. *BMJ* 2014;348:f7699.
16. Lenzer J. Majority of panellists on controversial new cholesterol guideline have current or recent ties to drug manufacturers. *BMJ* 2013;347:f6989.
17. Guidelines for the management of acute cervical spine and spinal cord injuries. Neurosurgery. March 2013 - Volume 72 - supplement 2, pp: 1–259
18. IMPACT-HAP Investigators Implementation of guidelines for management of possible multidrug-resistant pneumonia in intensive care: an observational, multicentre cohort study. Lancet On-Line: Jan 20th 2011
19. Bouri S, Shun-Shin MJ, Cole GD, *et al.* Meta-analysis of secure randomised controlled trials of β-blockade to prevent perioperative death in non-cardiac surgery of initiation of peri-operative beta blockers. *Heart* 2013 Jul 31. doi: 10.1136/heartjnl-2013-304262.
20. Laurie Barclay. Evidence underlying most guidelines may be questionable. January 21, 2014 Mayo Clinic Proc 2014;89:16-24.
21. Lenzer J. Why we can't trust clinical guidelines. *BMJ*. 2013;346:f3830. doi: 10.1136/bmj.f3830.
22. Edward Davies. Getting clinical guidelines right. *BMJ* 2013;347:f5733
23. Lenzer J, Hoffman JR, Furberg CD, *et al.* Ensuring the integrity of clinical practice guidelines: a tool for protecting patients. *BMJ* 2013;347:f5535.
24. Mabel Chew. How the BMJ selects guideline summaries for publication. *BMJ* 2013;347:f5536.
25. Edward Davies. Can you trust your clinical guidelines? *BMJ* 2013;346:f4003.

Pitfall No. 7

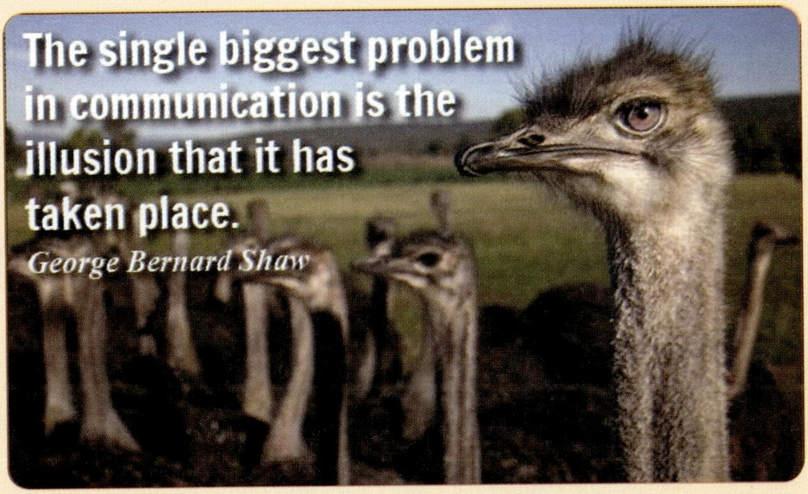
The single biggest problem in communication is the illusion that it has taken place.
George Bernard Shaw

Pitfall No. 7

Communication and Documentation

An effective tool to have a cooperative (& grateful) patient and family is to communicate. As it happens, this is also the most effective way to prevent future medicolegal issues.

The word communication is derived from the Latin words *'communis'* (noun) and '*communicare* (verb), and essentially means sharing of something, which in the medical context is sharing of knowledge and information.

Managing patients in the complex environment of ICU with its multidisciplinary teams requires the ability to skilfully communicate between the various teams as well as with patients and relatives. This forms one of the core non-technical skills required in ICUs. Most clinicians learn by modelling their teachers or senior colleagues. Personality also plays a role. With the world shrinking and becoming multicultural, language and culture too have an impact on our ability to communicate effectively. Literature suggests that training in communication skills enhances long-term skills and benefits both clinician and patient.[1] This has led to this type of training now being provided as a mandatory part of undergraduate and postgraduate medical training in some parts of the world. Although, this training is now part of the medical training curriculum in the western world, it continues to remain fragmented in countries such as India, despite there being an awareness of the need for the provision of this type of training.[2] But it shouldn't end once the training is completed. All healthcare professionals should keep striving to enhance personal effectiveness through their ability to communicate throughout their career.

Communication can be of various types: written, verbal, non-verbal e.g. gestures, body language etc. Written communication ensures that all events and decisions related to the patient are documented to allow for clear evidence of the decision making process. This is essential to allow statements to be written should the need arise especially in relation to medico legal issues. A study looking at 24 hour observation of written communication in ICU found that 18% of activities were not recorded in any form.[3] The same study also found that verbal communication between nurses and physicians was only documented in 37% of cases despite verbal communication being the commonest form of communication in ICU. Technically it is impossible to document every verbal communication as a lot of the communication is informal. But every attempt should be made to document relevant conversations between teams that impact patient care. Also, all interventions during patient care must be documented in the patient's notes.

Communication in ICU

Communication with Nurses

Teamwork in ICU between doctors and nurses needs to be well co-ordinated and any instructions for patient care must be clear to reduce any margin of error. A mutual respect for each other's skill and expertise also helps. Clear and concise documentation at ward rounds and during any patient related activity adds to maintaining patient safety. A study done in 2009 looked at specific elements of communication between nurses and clinicians and its impact on patient outcomes. As an example, timeliness of communication in this study was negatively associated with the prevalence of pressure ulcers. This suggests that clear and timely communication between teams has the capacity to improve patient outcomes.[4]

Not only is there a need for clinicians to communicate with the nursing staff during day to day activities, there is also a need to work synchronously during a crisis. Crisis management on ICU really brings all aspects of communication to the fore. This includes managing resources and allocating tasks, team working and situational awareness.[5] Multidisciplinary simulation is rapidly becoming the most sort after way to improving communication between teams in high stress situations.

Stressful situations on ICU can also lead to conflict between medical and nursing teams. Clarifying and resolving these issues at the earliest should take priority in order to avoid putting patients at risk. Above all, members of the team should be allowed to raise concerns in order to prevent adverse events.

Communication with Support Teams in ICU

Support teams provide much needed holistic care for the patient and as such should have clear instructions on what needs doing and what the plan for the patient is. This especially applies to the respiratory therapists and the physiotherapists. These teams also assist with ensuring that policies and protocols on the unit are followed and should be free to communicate with the medical and nursing teams if said policies are deviated from especially if there is a possibility of an adverse event.

Communication with Patients

Of all the communication in ICU, the one that is likely to cause the most impact is communication with patients and their families.

Many times in ICU, patient related discussions by the bedside are done without involving the conscious patient and the patients can feel left out of the discussion for their care as the discussions take place "above them" rather than "with them". One of the main reasons this happens is due to a large percentage of ICU patients being sedated and ventilated that we forget to include patients in discussions when they are awake and conscious and able to participate in these discussions. It should be routine practice to talk to awake and conscious patients and direct questions and discussions to them rather than only to the team. This will help build confidence in these patients during a very stressful episode in their lives.

Communication with Patients' Relatives

As a large proportion of patients in ICU are "unconscious" their families are the surrogates through which patient's wishes are elucidated and the clinical decisions discussed. In today's litigious world clear communication with families is becoming essential. Regular updates by the senior-most clinician is a simple way of ensuring that communication with families and relatives takes place.

One of the most stressful situations for both clinicians and patients' families is end of life discussions. It is not an uncommon occurrence in ICU and therefore, getting it right is essential. End of life conferences are the commonest way to have discussions with families. This not only allows the clinician to explain medical matters relating to the patient, but it also allows families the opportunity to raise questions and clarify issues. The mainstay of the language used to communicate during these discussions must be such that the families can understand and thus, needs to be clear and with the use of laymen terminology. This type of conference must necessarily be done without external interruptions. It is also important for clinicians to take the time to listen to relatives and families during these discussions. Most families struggle to make a decision regarding end of life care, which is many times interpreted as "ending the life" of a loved one. Supporting the families when difficult decisions need to be made will also help families accept realistic goals of treatment.[6] In order for the families to make a pragmatic decision a full and thorough discussion of what treatment modalities will be used and those which will not be, must be had with an emphasis on comfort measures and alleviation of pain. A paternalistic approach to family discussions must be avoided at all cost. Many times a single discussion will not be enough and repeat discussions will need to take place.

Along with verbal discussions written information e.g. bereavement brochures also help families to consolidate what is discussed.[7]

A clear strategy on how and what needs to be discussed will help the clinician with ensuring that all that needs discussing is discussed and consensus decisions are arrived at.

Empathy and a plan for open visiting hours for families with a loved one at end of life will provide a human touch to an otherwise clinical environment.

Communication with Junior Members of the Team e.g. Trainees / Residents

Trainees/residents, in a manner of speaking, are in their 'formative years' on ICU and learn mannerisms and nuances from their more senior colleagues and consultants. They are also most likely to be physically present on the unit out of hours. A study looking at cardio respiratory events in surgical ICU patients identified 33% communication errors by resident medical staff. Of all the communication errors that medical staff were involved in 77% were during late night shifts. By introducing a formal communication seminar the team managed to reduce error to 10%.[8] Emphasising the need for good communication within teams, patients and their families should thus form part of the day to day learning on ICU.

Trainees/residents are also involved in the handover process. Handovers are entirely about communicating and with most units around the world having some kind of shift working this becomes especially important. The trainees/residents need to ensure that not only the content in their handovers is factually accurate but a systematic approach should be followed to allow for no margin of error. This will also ensure that there is no missing information when one team hands over to another.

Communication outside ICU

Communication with the Primary Teams and Contributing Specialities

Depending on the type of unit one works in, the amount of communication and joint decision making varies. Closed units tend to cause slightly less conflict between the ICU and primary teams while there can be serious differences of opinion between teams working in open units. Clear chain of command, so to speak, must be established within units to reduce conflict between teams.

Primary teams should stay in the loop regarding their patients on ICU, not only so that they are clear about what has happened and what needs doing, but also because it keeps lines of communication open.

Discharging patients back to the primary teams after a stay on ICU requires clear communication, both written and verbal, to ensure continuity of care. Every effort must be made to ensure that this happens routinely for all patients. A concise summary of the ICU stay not only helps the primary team taking over care but also in the event of the patient requiring a repeat admission to ICU.

Similarly in the event of death of a patient on the unit, expected or otherwise, passing on the information to the primary team must take place.

Patients on ICU do tend to get opinions from various specialities. This in itself can lead to conflict and a power struggle between the admitting team, the intensivist, the speciality providing the opinion etc. It is vital that the decision making process has the patient as the focal point and all conflict is amicably resolved.

Conclusion

Effective communication between all multidisciplinary teams caring for patients on ICUs is required to ensure a cohesive and coordinated unit that keeps patient safety at its heart. Training in all aspects of communication skills early on in the career trajectory will help not only the members of the multidisciplinary teams but also the patients and their families.

References

1. Maguire P, Pitceathly C. Key communication skills and how to acquire them. *BMJ* 2002;325:697–700.
2. Chatterjee S, Choudhury N. Medical communication skills training in the Indian setting: Need of the hour. *Asian J Transfus Sci* 2011;5(1):8–10.
3. Donchin Y, Gopher D, Olin M, *et al.* A look into the nature and causes of human errors in the intensive care unit. *Crit Care Med* 1995; 23:294–300.
4. Manojlovich M, Antonakos CL, Ronis DL. Intensive Care Units, communication between nurses and physicians, and patients' outcomes. *Am J Crit Care* 2009;18(1):21–30.
5. Reader T, Flin R, Lauche K, *et al.* Non-technical skills in the intensive care unit. *Br J Anaesth* 2006;96(5):551–9.
6. Lautrette A, Darmon M, Megarbane B, *et al.* A communication strategy and brochure for relatives of patients dying in the ICU. *N Engl J Med* 2007;356:469–78.
7. Azoulay E, Pochard F, Chevret S, *et al.* Impact of a family information leaflet on effectiveness of information provided to family members of intensive care unit patients: a multicenter, prospective, randomized, controlled trial. *Am J Respir Crit Care Med* 2002;165:438–42.
8. Williams M, Hevelone N, Alban RF, *et al.* Measuring Communication in the Surgical ICU: Better Communication Equals Better Care. *J Am Coll Surg* 2010;210(1):17–22.

Pitfall No. 8

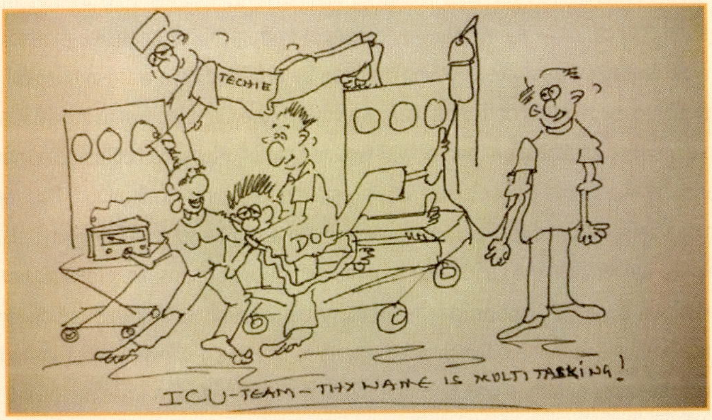

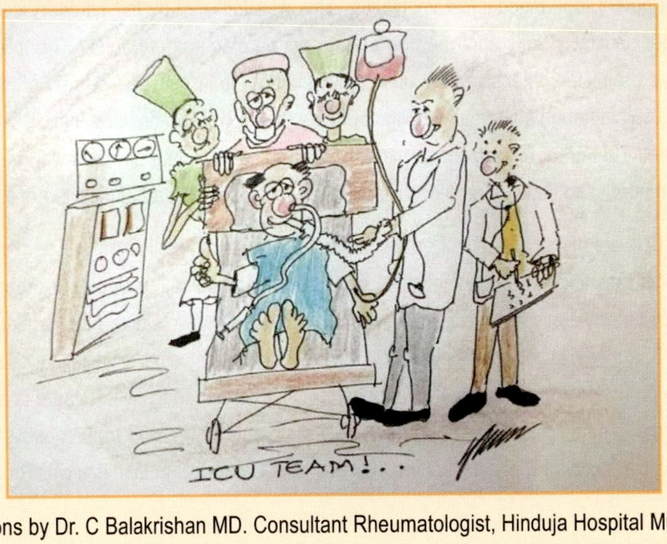

Cartoons by Dr. C Balakrishan MD. Consultant Rheumatologist, Hinduja Hospital Mumbai.

Pitfall No. 8

Inadequate Staffing

Intensive care medicine, as we know it today, hasn't evolved overnight. It has stemmed from a realization that critically ill patients would benefit from far more intensive monitoring and care in a dedicated area, unlike anything that can be provided on a ward in hospital. One of the simplest moves towards dedicated care was during the Crimean war in the 1850s, where more soldiers died of diseases than of war wounds, when Florence Nightingale moved the most seriously ill patients closer to the nursing station for closer monitoring.[1] This led to the creation of small dedicated recovery rooms which remained as such till the polio epidemic. It was the polio epidemic in the 1950s that saw the introduction of positive pressure ventilators with the wards becoming known as "respiratory care units". It was this advancement in mechanical ventilation that led the Scandinavians to use this technique in a variety of other respiratory diseases and thus was born the modern era of Intensive Care, revolving around its most potent tool, mechanical ventilation. This was followed by the coronary care units and other speciality units such as burns and post cardiac surgery units.[2] The late 1950s saw multidisciplinary intensive care units (ICUs) spring up in the US. The rest of the world followed suit although some developing countries took a while to develop their ICUs. In the 1960s and 70s, great organizational strides were made in setting up ICUs with personnel skilled in managing patients requiring mechanical ventilation as part of their therapy.

Today, ICUs are highly dependent on their infrastructure, technological as well as personnel, to provide care tailored to the individual needs of the critically ill patients. In order to run efficiently is a resource intensive process, not just in terms of workforce but also financially. In the US, the cost is approximately $3500 each day for intensive care[3] while in the UK each bed day on ICU is approximately £1700.[4] On the other hand in India, where there is a dearth of systematic data on cost implications of ICU stay, data from 2005 from a public-private sector cancer hospital suggests that the total cost of ICU care per patient day was Rs. 12,000 (approximately US $273), much less than the developed world[5] while that in a private hospital is much higher. Using data from 2010 in a private hospital, the daily cost of an ICU bed varied from Rs 4,600-10,400/- per day. Depending on disease and duration of ICU stay, this direct ICU bed charge accounted from 7 to 74% of the total bill (mean 28% median 22%) for medical or emergency patients and was only about 5% in elective surgical patients.[5]

The situation in the developing world in some respects is entirely different to that in the developed one. While ICUs are well established in the developed world and the focus in on standardization e.g. in the UK, in the developing world e.g. India the focus still remains on developing an infrastructure for ICU to firstly be able to meet the needs of an ever growing population. Thus focus on standardization and staffing becomes a completely secondary issue. Having said that, ignoring the issue of adequate staffing and resource allocation will eventually be to the detriment of the patient.

Over the years, the literature has suggested that the organizational structure of an intensive care unit may have bearing on the clinical outcomes for patients. This has led to an attempt at standardization of facilities and care in ICUs although, worldwide variability in the organization and provision of critical care services still exist.

The Indian Society of Critical Care Medicine has played a pivotal role in developing guidelines for ICU design and delivery of care, something that was first published nearly 10 years ago. In the UK, the first edition of the guidelines for the provision of Intensive Care services was published in April 2015 by the Intensive Care society.[4] The mainstay of this document is the Core Standards for ICUs which were published by the Faculty of Intensive care (FICM) in 2013,[6] which describe in great detail delivery of intensive care services.

Staffing

Intensive Care Units comprise of high intensity level of care with all levels of staff having to function under undue stress which also carries the burden of high emotional cost for its workforce. This is associated with conflicts within teams and a high burn out rate. Optimum staffing for an ICU is still unclear although common sense dictates that better the staffing levels the better the overall outcomes for both patients and staff.

Medical

Intensive Care teams and patient care are generally led by the Consultant Intensivist. Evidence supports the presence of a Consultant Intensivist with improved outcomes for patients in ICU.[7] These consultants can have a variety of base speciality experience e.g.

general medicine, respiratory medicine, anesthetics, cardiology, emergency medicine and general surgery. This tends to vary from country to country, for e.g. in India general medicine is the most common base speciality for intensivists while in the UK it's anesthetics. Whatever the base speciality, consultants in ICU provide the continuity of care that is vital and bring a certain level of expertise dependant on their base speciality. Level of experience for Consultant Intensivists, in countries where the speciality is manned by consultants without the requisite official qualifications, is defined by their experience and the number of years spent within the speciality. As an example, in India, the experience is quantified as a minimum 3 years' experience in a Level 2 ICU, and 5 years' experience in a Level 3 ICU.[8]

Work patterns in ICU vary from unit to unit and country to country. A study in 2011 suggested that 5 day continuous working with a break over the weekends versus a 2 week rotation, was associated with reduced consultant burn out and not only did it provide continuity of care, this type of working did not worsen clinical outcomes.[9] The European Society of Intensive Care Medicine (ESICM) on the other hand recommends that ICU care should be delivered by trained intensivists 24 hours a day 7 days a week.[10] Although, in an ideal world having the ICU staffed just by intensivists is the way forward, given the dearth of intensivists in this rapidly advancing speciality this remains an aspirational dream for many units around the world.

No specific consultant to patient ratio exists for India but the recommended consultant to patient ratio, by the FICM and the ESICM is between 1:8–1:14.[6,12] These consultants are required to conduct structured multi-disciplinary ward rounds daily to plan the day to day care of the patients on the unit.

Every unit needs a Lead who has the managerial responsibility for the unit. Thus, there must be a designated Head of Unit / Department or Lead for the ICU.

Along with consultants ICUs are staffed with junior medical staff e.g. trainees or residents. The ICU environment should be conducive to providing the trainees with training and experience and the trainees should actively participate in the day to day working of the unit and delivery of patient care. The recommendation for trainee doctors to patient ratio in India is 1:10 – 1:14,[11] while it is 1:8 patients in the UK.[6]

Nursing

The difference between medical and nurse staffing, is the direct hands on care that needs to be provided by the nursing staff. Thus, there are always way more nurses in the ICU than medical staff. But the nurse to patient ratio varies tremendously between not just units but also countries. Some units are successful in implementing the 1:1 nurse to patient ratio while others simply can't afford this luxury. Highly specialized units with manpower intense technologies such as extracorporeal membrane oxygenation (ECMO) do have nurse patient ratios of 2:1, at least in the initial phase of treatment.

What then should be the ideal nurse patient ratios for ICUs to aspire to? This depends on the complexity of patients. Level 3 care is defined as patients requiring advanced respiratory care or basic respiratory care with 2 additional organs being supported, while Level 2 care is defined as patients requiring single organ support or more detailed monitoring. In the UK, the recommendation is for 1:1 nurse patient ratio for direct care of Level 3 patients while a 1:2 nurse patient ratio is acceptable for direct care of Level 2 patients.[4]

A study of 69 ICUs in the US, published in 2014, concluded that a lower bed-to-nurse ratio was associated with a lower annual ICU mortality.[3] Investing in adequate numbers of skilled nursing staff on ICU will go a long way to improve patient outcomes.

Respiratory Technicians/Therapists

Respiratory Therapists form part of the intensive care team in some countries like the US, India etc. Their role extends to anything related to managing artificial airways including providing vital assistance during procedures like percutaneous tracheostomies, bronchoscopies, intubations etc. Currently, no definitive recommendations for staffing exist for respiratory therapists but a study published in 2013[13] suggests a respiratory therapist to patient ratio of 1:10 improves utilization than the earlier recommendation of 1:14.[14]

Physiotherapists

Evidence to suggest early rehabilitation of patients in intensive care to reduce post intensive care morbidity is mounting and physiotherapists play a vital role in achieving better outcomes for patients in this regard. Most ICUs tend to use physiotherapists from the hospital pool. The ESICM recommends the availability of a trained physiotherapist per 5 beds 24/7.[7]

Dieticians

Critically ill patients require their nutritional needs to be monitored and met via the most appropriate route possible. Dieticians can assist with this process and should be available to ICUs to help tailor the provision of nutritional support to the patient's needs.

Microbiologists

Microbiology ward rounds in ICU help with the effective and prompt management of infections and also assist with antibiotic stewardship.

Pharmacists

The role of the critical care pharmacist has expanded over the years and now forms an integral part of the multidisciplinary team on ICU. As they have in-depth knowledge of pharmacotherapy and pharmacokinetics they assist clinicians with decision making by providing drug information and also in monitoring drug safety. They should be available to consult ideally 24/7 but as a minimum during working hours.

Organization and Infrastructure

Intensive care units are heavily dependent on technology for the provision of patient care and monitoring. Over the years technology has advanced and moved from the bulky equipment of the yesteryears to the much smaller models we see now. Not just that, the innovation in the type of monitoring has also come leaps and bounds. Information technology too has made ingress into ICUs and now it is not only possible to see laboratory results and imaging at a patient's bedside but also there are now paperless units in the world with all documentation being done electronically. With Robotic telepresence gaining momentum are the ICUs of the future going to be mechanized? This is something only time will tell. For now though, setting up an ICU requires a fair bit of investment especially if the latest in technology is to be installed and if the best infrastructure is to be implemented. But once that's done there are just the ongoing costs of maintaining the equipment and the infrastructure.

Handover

Intensive care units work on some form of shift patterns for its staff. This necessitates a patient handover from one shift to another. Patient safety depends on the quality of handovers between various members of staff to prevent adverse events. Although, handovers have been done for decades, every unit seems to have its own way of doing the handovers. Some units have a joint handover at change of shift with the medical and nursing teams present, yet some have nurses handing over to nurses and doctors handing over to doctors and no joint communication between the two teams. Handovers to the ward based teams when the patient is discharged from ICU also tend to be a bit hit and miss.

Critically ill patents are complex and therefore, structured and standardized handovers with the multidisciplinary team are now recommended for all handovers. Medical handovers in the presence of the unit consultant and the senior nurse/sister of the unit improve the quality of handovers. Variations in the type of handovers include a "sit down" handover with the multi-disciplinary team or a "walk around" handover. No one system is perfect and every unit will need to adapt and modify the process in order to achieve the best outcome for patients.

Deteriorating Patient on the Ward

Intensive care units have always participated, in some shape or form, in resuscitating the acutely unwell patient on the hospital wards. They are called by different names in different countries e.g. Rapid Response Teams in India, Medical Emergency Teams in Australia, and Cardiac Arrest Teams in the UK etc. While it's a good idea to have a team to respond to emergencies, in some cases it might be a case of too little too late. Recently the remit and scope of intensive care has widened to include the deteriorating patient on the wards in hospital, in some countries. The belief is that if recognized earlier and with appropriate early intervention patient outcomes can be improved. And who best placed to provide this kind of long reach service other than the intensive care teams. This has led to the formation of the "outreach" teams which comprise of staff with intensive care skills that advice the wards on the management of the acutely deteriorating patient. Most hospitals in the western world now have some kind of early warning score to facilitate the identification of the deteriorating patient so that the appropriate response can be triggered. The outreach teams work in conjunction with the Rapid response teams and the like, thus providing much needed support in an emergency.

Protocols and Policies

In order to have a seamless way of delivering care on ICUs standard practice needs to have embedded protocols and policies in order to improve patient outcomes. These policies should be such that there is enough leeway to allow for inter patient variability and thus provide patient centred care. This has been discussed at length in the chapter Pitfall No 6.

Conclusion

Intensive Care Units need both, an excellent infrastructure and adequate staff. While the infrastructure is a one off cost, the staff that forms the backbone of any good unit remains an expensive commodity. In order to ensure good clinical outcomes investing in appropriately trained staff and ensuring a good staff to patient ratio is paramount.

References

1. Vincent JL. Critical care – where have we been and where are we going? *Crit Care* 2013;17(Suppl 1):S2.
2. Robert Rodriguez. Demystifying critical care. *West J Med* 2001;175(6):366–67.
3. Checkley W, Martin GS, Brown SM, *et al*. Structure, process and annual intensive care unit mortality across 69 centers: United States Critical Illness and Injury Trials Group Critical Illness Outcomes Study (USCIITG-CIOS). *Crit Care Med* 2014; 42(2):344–56.
4. ICS. Guidelines for the Provision of Intensive Care Services. Edition 1 / 2015

5. Farhad Kapadia, Atul P. Kulkarni, JV Divatia India: Where Have We Been. (pp 33-38) In ICU Resource Allocation in the New Millennium: International Perspective in ICU Resource Allocation in the New Millennium. Will We Say "No"? (Editor David W. Crippen) Springer (ISBN 978-1-4614-3865-6, ISBN 978-1-4614-3866-3 (eBook))
6. FICM. Core Standards for Intensive Care Units. Edition 1 / 2013
7. Pronovost PJ, Angus DC, Dorman T, *et al.* Physician staffing patterns and clinical outcomes in critically ill patients: a systematic review. *JAMA* 2002;288:2151–62.
8. Critical Care Delivery in Intensive Care Units in India: Defining the Functions, Roles and Responsibilities of a Consultant intensivist. Recommendations of the Indian Society of Critical Care Medicine Committee on Defining the Functions, Roles and Responsibilities of a Consultant intensivist. Guidelines Committee ISCCM.
9. Ali NA, Hammersley J, Hoffman SP, *et al.* Continuity of care in intensive care units a cluster-randomized trial of intensivist staffing. *Am J Respir Crit Care Med* 2011;184(7):803–08.
10. Valentin A, Ferdinande P; ESICM Working Group on Quality Improvement. Recommendations on basic requirements for intensive care units: structural and organizational aspects. *Intensive Care Med* 2011;37(10):1575–87.
11. ICU Planning and Designing in India – Guidelines 2010. Guidelines Committee ISCCM.
12. Ward NS1, Afessa B, Kleinpell R, *et al.* Members of Society of Critical Care Medicine Taskforce on ICU Staffing. Intensivist/patient ratios in closed ICUs: a statement from the Society of Critical Care Medicine Taskforce on ICU Staffing. *Crit Care Med* 2013;41(2):638–45.
13. Parker AM, Liu X, Harris AD, *et al.* Respiratory therapy organizational changes are associated with increased respiratory care utilization. *Respiratory Care* 2013;58(3):438–49.
14. Mathews P, Drumheller L, Carlow JJ. Respiratory care manpower issues. *Crit Care Med* 2006;34(3 Suppl):S32–S45.

Pitfalls 9

CASE SCENARIO

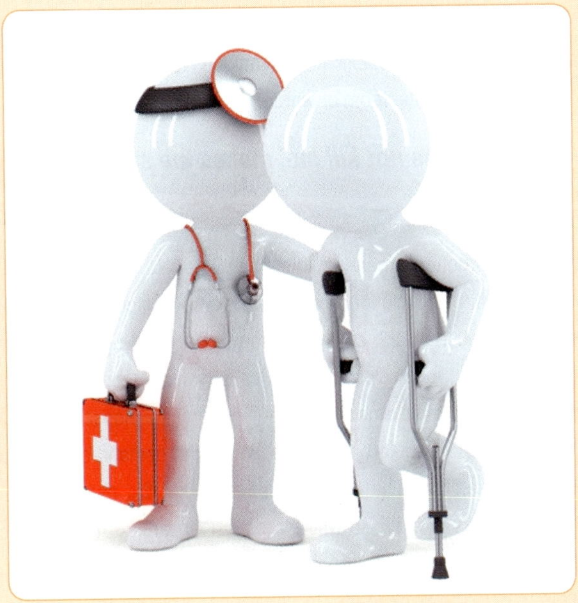

Scenario 1: Patient recovers over the next 3-4 weeks. The sedation is withdrawn, and the patient is weaned off life support. He is observed in ICU and later transferred to the ward. He is weak and poorly mobile and is advised to rest for a few days. He is then discharged home. After discharge, he is still weak and breathless on mobilization. He tends to be forgetful and "is not his old self". He is then started on a physiotherapy program. It takes another 3 months to become physically functional and independent and another three months to go back to his job.

What was the Pitfall?

Pitfall No. 9

Delayed & Inadequate Rehabilitation

The Pitfall was not implementing rehabilitation techniques during and after the critical illness, either in the ICU or in the hospital room or wards.

What does not kill me, makes me stronger.

– Friedrich Nietzsche 1888

The muscles are the forgotten organs of Intensive Care. No aspect of care is aimed at preserving or strengthening muscle function. Yet from an evolutionary perspective, we have multiple organ-systems such as the circulation, the blood, the lungs, and the neurological system to primarily serve the muscles. The survival advantage conferred by locomotion is what drove the evolution of these organ-systems. If one has to choose a physiological state most akin to critical illness, it would be exercise, where the demand on the organ-systems of the body increase manifold. The main difference is that the muscles are the oxygen and energy hungry organs in exercise while in critical illness the muscles are quiescent, but there is a general increase in metabolic demand, including the immune-inflammatory system. Muscles respond to work loads. In conditions of disuse they atrophy, while with heavy exercise, especially resistance exercise, they hypertrophy. All of exercise training is built around this principle; gradually increase the load on muscles and they become stronger. Physiotherapy is essentially controlled exercise for those recovering from illness, injury or surgery. Table 1 gives a brief comparison of the demands on the physiological organ-systems due to critical illness and exercise. If one spends some time thinking about the numbers in this table, it should become apparent that the demands of exercise are in a different order of magnitude from the basal requirements and also significantly more than the requirements during a critical illness. Of course exercise sessions are much shorter than a critical illness, and unlike a critically ill patient, the athlete always has the option of stopping

Table 1. Oxygenation, Perfusion and Cardio-Respiratory variables at rest, in Critical Illness and during Exercise (Figures taken from Guyton's Textbook of Physiology)

Physiological Variable (unit)	Normal at Rest	Hyper-metabolic Critical Illness	Peak Exercise (young fit male)	Elite Marathoner
O2 Utilization (mL/min)	250	400-500	3500-4000	5000
Tissue Blood Flow (mL/100 gm muscle/min)	3.6		90	
Cardiac Output (L/min)	5	10-20	20-30	35-40
Minute Ventilation (L/Min)	7-9	10-20	100-110	
Alveolar O_2 diffusion rate (mL/min/ mmHg a-A O_2 difference)	23		48	65-80

and immediately decreasing the metabolic demand. Still, these numbers make one question the belief that multi-organ failure (MOF) is simply due to an energy deficit. It appears that the ability of the body to supply oxygen is greater than the demands critical illness places on it. Something else is happening. One view is that MOF is a failure to produce energy, Adenosine Tri-Phosphate (ATP), despite an adequate oxygen supply due to mitochondrial dysfunction. An alternative view is that MOF is primarily a cellular failure despite an adequate energy supply. (An analogy is that a car may not work for multiple reasons despite having a full tank of petrol and similarly a mobile phone may not work despite having a fully charged battery). Yet another view is that MOF is a protective mechanism. The cells produce just enough ATP and energy to maintain cellular integrity, but not enough to do any additional work or function. It is the human version of hibernation. In conditions of scarcity, certain animals such as bears have the ability to turn their metabolism down to bare sustenance levels. Waking such an animal up and increasing its metabolism will actually decrease the chance of survival. Another analogy is that of a wounded soldier, who opts to lie down and heal, rather than die by going back into battle. Regardless of the underlying mechanism, the nerves and muscles too are not spared in this cellular failure. Some forms of intensive care unit acquired weakness are due to cellular alterations of the muscle and nerve.

It is now recognized that ICU acquired weakness is a major and common sequel of critical illness.[1] During critical illness, up to 25-50% of patients will have some residual weakness, and among patients with severe prolonged sepsis and multi-organ failure requiring ventilation, the incidence of weakness approaches 100%. This weakness may be due to a variety of neuromuscular problems sometimes called Critical Illness Polyneuropathy and Critical Illness Myopathy (CIP-CIM). Table 2 shows the various forms of this illness. The diagnosis is

Table 2. Generalized neuromuscular disorders associated with critical illness[1]

	Incidence	Clinical features	Electrophysiological findings	Serum creatine kinase	Muscle biopsy	Prognosis
Polyneuricpathy						
Critical illness polyneuropathy	Common	Flaccid limbs, respiratory weakness	Axonal degeneration of motor and sensory fibres	Nearly normal	Denervation atrophy	Variable
Neuromuscular transmission defect						
Transient neuromuscular blockade	Common with neuromuscular blocking agents	Flaccid limbs, respiratory weakness	Abnormal repetitive nerve stimulation studies	Normal	Normal	Good
Critical illness myopathy						
Thick-filament myopathy	Common with steroids, neuromuscular blocking agents, and sepsis	Flaccid limbs, respiratory weakness	Abnormal spontaneous activity	Mildly elevated	Loss of thick (myosin) filament	Good
Acute myopathy with scattered necrosis	Common	Flaccid limbs, respiratory weakness	Myopathy	Mildly or moderately raised	Scattered necrosis	Variable
Acute myopathy with diffuse necrosis (necrotizing myopathy of intensive care)	Rare	Flaccid weakness, myoglobinuria	Severe myopathy	Greatly raised, myoglobinuria	Marked necrosis	Poor
Disuse (cachectic) myopathy	Common	Muscle wasting	Normal	Normal	Normal or type II fibre atrophy	Variable
Rhabdomyolysis	Rare	Flaccid limbs	Near normal	Markedly elevated (myoglobinuria)	Normal or mild necrosis	Good
Combined polyneuropathy and myopathy	Common	Flaccid limbs, respiratory weakness	Indicative of combined polyneuropathy and myopathy	Variable	Denervation atrophy and myopathy	Variable

Modified from Bolton,27 by permission of Springer

based on clinical features and occasionally needs electrophysiology and biopsy. Obviously rapidly treating the illness and limiting its severity and duration is the best way to prevent CIP-CIM. As of now the only other technique which is shown to be beneficial in limiting the severity and hastening the recovery from CIP-CIM is physiotherapy and mobilization. Tight sugar control too may be beneficial, but is not currently recommended in view of its negative impact on 90-day mortality in the NICE-SUGAR study.[2]

The "Post Intensive Care Syndrome"

ICU acquired weakness is not the only problem faced by survivors of a critical illness. In fact, there are so many long term problems faced by survivors that it is sometimes called the Post Intensive Care Syndrome.[3] Survivors of acute respiratory distress syndrome (ARDS) have residual functional disability at even 5 years.[4] Some of this disability is due to permanent lung damage and fibrosis. There has been a report of a survivor of ARDS needing a lung transplant due to the extensive fibrosis and honeycombing that occurred in the fibroproliferative phase of the disease. This functional disability is not only because of fibrotic changes in the lung, but also has a large muscular component. A significant percentage of patients with acute renal failure (ARF) progress to dialysis dependent chronic renal failure (CRF) due to renal loss.[5] They have a higher incidence of both cardiovascular and cerebrovascular events compared to matched controls.[6] Besides these major organ dysfunctions, there are lists of neurological problems too in the survivors of severe critical illness. The Post Traumatic Stress Disorder is common and may occur in up to 50% of ICU survivors.[7] More worryingly, cognitive decline and loss are frequently seen.[8,9] Recently, depression has been recognized as another consequence of critical illness occurring with an equal frequency of about 30% in those with and without a prior diagnosis of depression. It often manifests with physical-somatic rather than emotional or cognitive manifestations.[10] Patients who were frail on admission had worse outcomes compared to non-frail patients, again presumably because of the reduced muscular and cardiac reserve.[11] Finally, as a result of all these problems, survivors have a higher mortality than the general population.[12] There have also been multiple reports of psychological and stress related problems in the families of the survivors.

Many strategies have been used to try and limit these problems. These include early nutrition, anabolic steroids, minimizing sedation, spontaneous awakening trials, using spontaneous modes of ventilation, early tracheotomy and nurse-led follow-up. Most of them have been unsuccessful. Neuro-psychiatric services are rarely offered to survivors of critical illness and may be beneficial. The only technique that has shown promise is physical therapy and mobilization. This can be done when on the mechanical ventilator in the ICU, as an in-patient, in a rehabilitation center, or as an out-patient. It consists of two basic components, neuro muscular and cardiovascular. The basic three components of exercise are strength, power and endurance. Technically, strength refers to the ability to overcome resistance and is a reflection of the amount of functioning contractile protein (actin-myosin) in the muscles. Power refers to the ability to sustain the work and is a reflection of the cellular ATP production and reserve, which in turn depends on both the mitochondrial function and the adequacy of the enzymes of the glycolytic pathway. Endurance refers to the ability of the body to keep replenishing the muscle energy stores and is a direct reflection of the cardiovascular reserves. The physiotherapy program should ensure all three components are trained. In addition, the program should use exercises that improve other aspects of motor function such as agility, balance and coordination. Another aspect of physiology to consider is the "Stress-Adaptation-Exhaustion" model. The body initially responds to any stressful muscular load by adapting and becoming stronger. Beyond a point however the response will be an exhausted response with worsening of strength, or with an injury. The program should be of an intensity to ensure adaptive improvement in performance, but not so intense as to precipitate an exhausted response.

The beneficial role of physiotherapy for ICU patients has previously been demonstrated in the post hospital setting, as well as during the ICU phase.[13]

A recent observational study[14] selectively evaluated patients with electro-physiologically confirmed CIP-CIM. The functional assessment was impressively detailed and included motor, cognitive and to some degree aerobic status with a 6 min walk test. The actual program was complex, individually designed and consisted of kinesiotherapy, electrotherapy, functional occupational therapy, daily activities training and psychosocial support. Overall the program showed benefit in functional status, muscle power and walking ability. The benefit was more marked if the program was started earlier in the recovery phase of the illness. Another "minimized controlled trial"[15] evaluated the effect of a supervised aerobic exercise rehabilitation program in ICU patients. The intervention group followed a moderate intensity exercise for 8 weeks and showed benefit at 9 weeks. A meta-analysis of 14 studies[16] looked at RCTs in which Physical Function (PF) was an endpoint, regardless of which intervention was being evaluated. Only exercise or physiotherapy was associated with improved PF. No other drug, therapeutic strategy or medical supervision had a positive impact on PF. It is worth noting that in most of these studies, all patients gain varying degrees of functional recovery. Those enrolled in an intensive physiotherapy and rehabilitation program primarily improve faster than control subjects. Lastly, a recent observational study looked at physiotherapy in mechanically ventilated patients and found that despite adequate physiotherapy staff, the minority actually got early mobilization while on mechanical ventilation. Most of this was mobilization in the bed and passive sitting. Just 3% of mobilization on mechanical ventilation involved standing or walking. The two biggest barriers were intubation and deep sedation. Other perceived barriers limiting mobilization were inotropes, femoral lines, pulmonary artery catheters, respiratory rate, agitation and weakness. They did note that increased muscle strength at ICU discharge was associated with early mobilization during mechanical ventilation and also associated with increased hospital and 90 day survival.[17]

Conclusion

Critical illness is followed by profound weakness and other organ system dysfunction. Physiotherapy and rehabilitation programs should be started as soon as possible during the critical illness and even when on mechanical ventilation rather than after ICU and hospital discharge. The program should include improvement of motor function, as well as improving cognitive, neuropsychiatric and occupational outcomes.

References

1. Nicola Latronico, Charles F Bolton. Critical illness polyneuropathy and myopathy: a major cause of muscle weakness and paralysis. *Lancet Neurol* 2011;10:931–41.
2. Intensive versus Conventional Glucose Control in Critically Ill Patients. The NICE-SUGAR Study Investigators. *N Engl J Med* 2009;360:1283–97.
3. Needham DM, Davidson J, Cohen H, *et al.* Improving long-term outcomes after discharge from intensive care unit: report from a stakeholders' conference. *Crit Care Med* 2012;40:502–09.
4. Herridge MS, Tansey CM, Matt. A, *et al.* Functional disability 5 years after acute respiratory distress syndrome. *N Engl J Med* 2011;364:1293–304.
5. RENAL Trial *N Engl J Med* 2009;361(17):1627-38. VA/NIH ATN Trial *N Engl J Med* 2008;359(1):7–20.
6. Yende S, Linde-Zwirble W, Mayr F, *et al.* Risk of cardiovascular events in survivors of severe sepsis. *Am J Respir Crit Care Med* 2014;189:1065–74.
7. Davydow DS, Gifford JM, Desai SV, *et al.* Post-traumatic stress disorder in general intensive care unit survivors: a systematic review. *Gen Hosp Psychiatry* 2008;30: 421–34.
8. Pandharipande PP, Girard TD, Jackson JC, *et al.* Long-term cognitive impairment after critical illness. *N Engl J Med* 2013;369:1306–16.
9. Iwashyna TJ, Ely EW, Smith DM, *et al.* Long-term cognitive impairment and functional disability among survivors of severe sepsis. *JAMA* 2010;304:1787–94.
10. BRAIN-ICU study. *Lancet Respir Med* 2014;2:369–79.
11. Bagshaw SM, Stelfox HT, McDermid RC *et al.* Association between frailty and short- and long-term outcomes among critically ill patients: a multicentre prospective cohort study. *CMAJ* 2014;186:E95–102.
12. Wieske L, Dettling-Ihnenfeldt DS, Verhamme C, *et al.* Impact of ICU-acquired weakness on post-ICU physical functioning: a follow-up study. *Critical Care* 2015;19:196.
13. Adler J, Malone D. Early Mobilization in the Intensive Care Unit: A Systematic Review. *Cardiopulm Phys Ther J* 2012;23:5–13.

14. Novak P, Vidmar G, Kuret Z, *et al.* Rehabilitation of critical illness polyneuropathy and myopathy patients: an observational study. *Int J Rehabilitation Res* 2011;34:336–42.
15. Batterham AM, Bonner S, Wright J, *et al.* Effect of supervised aerobic exercise rehabilitation on physical fitness and quality-of-life in survivors of critical illness: an exploratory minimized controlled trial (PIX study). *Br J Anaesthes* 2104.
16. Calvo-Ayala E. Interventions to improve the physical function of ICU survivors. *Chest* 2013;144:1469–80.
17. The TEAM Study Investigators. Early mobilization and recovery in mechanically ventilated patients in the ICU: a bi-national, multi-centre, prospective cohort study. *Critical Care* 2015;19:81.

Pitfalls 10

CASE SCENARIO

Scenario 2a: Two days later, the immediate family members come to the intensive care unit (ICU) and inform the doctors that the patient has a history of chronic obstructive pulmonary disease (COPD), Alzheimer's with aspiration and minimal mobility for 3-6 months. Tracheal aspirate is positive for malignant cells. Further imaging suggests metastatic disease. Inotropes and ventilation are continued. Patient then becomes anuric and dialysis is started. Patient then suffers 3 episodes of cardiac arrest requiring cardiopulmonary resuscitation (CPR). He is resuscitated each time. The 4th time after half hearted attempts at resuscitation (the so called slow code) the family is informed that the patient has passed away despite all possible medical efforts.

Scenario 2b: Patient remains in refractory multiple organ failure (MOF). The family asks if therapy can be limited or withdrawn. They are informed that it is not possible as it is a form of euthanasia and hence against the law. However, they are "unofficially" told that they can insist on taking him home, and the hospital will record it as a "Left Against Medical Advice" (LAMA) situation. A local practitioner, at the request of the family, arrives at the hospital, connects the patient to an AMBU bag and he is transported out of hospital. The team is later informed that the patients has passed away but are given no details as to whether he was extubated terminally at home.

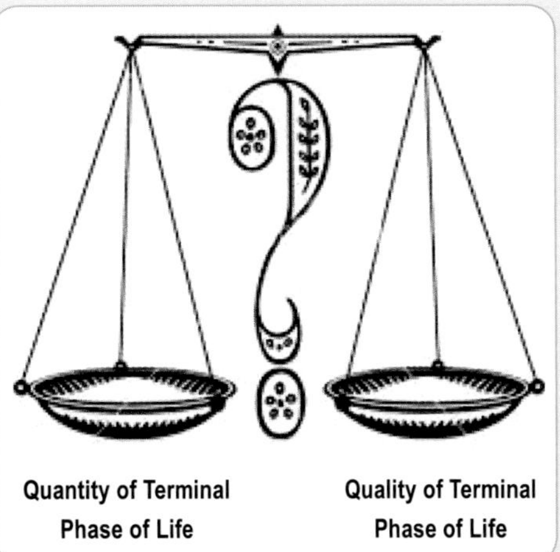

What is the Pitfall?

Pitfall No. 10

No End of Life (EoL) Care Plan

The pitfalls are:

a) Failure to clearly communicate the terminal nature of the disease and

b) Subsequent failure to proactively make an End of Life (EoL) plan.

As George Washington lay on his deathbed, doctors applied a dried-beetle mixture to his skin to induce blistering; gave him a mercury compound to clear his digestive system; and took five pints of blood from his veins. Before he died later that day, he was treated by three eminent physicians who were taking heroic measures they thought appropriate in trying to save a former president.

The above care is patently absurd to modern minds. Yet many intensive care units (ICUs) continue to practice a variation of this. Substitute induced blistering, digestive clearance and bloodletting with vasoactive medication, intubation and mechanical ventilation and dialysis and we have the modern form of the above treatment. The underlying pitfall is the same today as it was in George Washington's: A failure of the physician to communicate the terminal nature of the illness, and to go through the motions of offering care, which is clearly futile. Communication is the key to ensuring that the terminal phase of a disease in the ICU is as comfortable as possible.

The first step in initiating an end of life (EoL) plan is to ensure that the disease has become irreversible. It is important to clearly separate out severity from irreversibility. A patient in profound multi organ failure (MOF) on life support following a road traffic accident or severe malaria is potentially salvageable, regardless of the severity of the MOF. A patient with end stage malignancy, liver, lung or heart disease is not likely to benefit from a stint of life support in ICU as the underlying condition cannot be reversed by ICU therapies. At some point MOF from a reversible cause becomes irreversible. We currently have no way to determine that point, so one errs on the side of continuing life support rather than considering some limitation of care. If the pupils become fixed and the patient becomes totally unresponsive solely due to MOF, it is probably terminal. Similarly, if the support is rapidly escalating or the lactate worsening, in the face of optimal or maximal treatment, it is probably terminal. If there is a doubt about the terminal nature of the disease, it is better to seek a professional consensus before initiating an EoL care plan.

In modern ICUs, once the terminal nature of the disease is established, EoL care is based on changing focus. The emphasis is to ensure comfort and absence of distress. One can stop other death delaying interventions and therapies when there is consensus that they are not serving any purpose for the patient.

If there has been clear communication as to what treatment is to be provided and what is not, the treating team can ensure comfort measures are delivered and also ensure that other unnecessary interventions are not implemented. This requires open and transparent communication well before the terminal phase. In an ICU setting, this communication is done between the treating physicians and the family members. Not infrequently, the patient has expressed a desire to limit treatment to the family, but the family is unsure how to proceed once the terminal phase has arrived. They need to be reassured that limiting treatment to comfort measures is acceptable and is indeed the correct thing to do. They need to be told that their relative is no longer in a position to express his or her wishes for terminal care and it is therefore, their responsibility to act on behalf of the patient, specifically if the patient has expressed these wishes earlier. When there is no prior communication, the physician needs to explain that the relatives should not decide what they feel is correct, but to decide on the basis of what they think the patient would have wanted. This communication has to be repeatedly done, as it is very difficult for the relatives to grasp the whole picture the first time around.

Obviously this brings in a whole series of ethical as well as socio-cultural issues. Each social-cultural-religious group has certain beliefs as to the right way of handling these situations, but the physician must be guided primarily by the medical ethics and not blindly follow the dictates of others. The four principles of medical ethics are Beneficence, Non-Maleficence, Autonomy and Social or Distributive Justice

---

Physicians must be guided primarily by the medical ethics of Beneficence, Non-Maleficence, Autonomy and Social or Distributive Justice.

Beneficence: Medical decisions must be made in the best interest of the patient. This sounds obvious, but as earlier chapters have shown, many ineffective therapies are routinely used in ICU patients, with the hope that there will be some benefit.

Non-Maleficence: First, Do No Harm; *"Primum non nocere"* This implies that the physician must take all care and precautions to ensure that harm does not befall a patient due to the treatment being offered. There is a somewhat similar term Non-Malfiecence which implies absence of bad intent. From the medical and ethical perspective, it is not enough not to have bad intent. Even with good intent, the physician must ensure that the treatments offered do not cause harm.

Autonomy: The patients decisions are supreme. Neither the physician nor the family as surrogate decision makers can override these decisions as long as the physician is convinced they are made with a sound mind.

Social or Distributive Justice: No one individual patient or family can claim right to all the resources and beds in the ICU. The ICU resources have to be distributed in a way with ensures they are compatible with social justice and equality.

These are not black and white situations and the same act can be viewed as ethical or unethical by different observers. For example, inserting an endotracheal tube in a clearly futile situation can be viewed as beneficial as it permits ventilation and oxygenation, but also considered maleficent as it induces significant pain and discomfort. Similarly, prolonging a patient's death by 5-10 days by artificial means such as ventilation and dialysis at the request of the relatives can be seen as respecting their autonomy, but allowing deserving patients to miss out on much needed intensive care therapy due to blocking of beds and leading to potentially avoidable mortality does not ensure social justice.

The key to good EoL care is communication. Ideally, this should be discussed prior to ICU transfer, preferably by the primary consultant, and if possible prior to hospitalization. The following are the issues that should be discussed. The first is that in terminal situations we do not need to transfer all dying patients to ICU, intubate, ventilate, dialyze and do CPR. There are various options for limitation of care. The terms used most often are withhold (WH) or withdraw (WD). The former is used when treatment is no longer increased, but continued at the existing level, while the latter is the stopping of all medications that do not contribute to comfort. Two other common terms are Do Not Intubate (DNI) and Do Not Resuscitate

---

The key to good EoL care is communication.

Two common terms are Do Not Intubate (DNI) and Do Not Resuscitate (DNR).

(DNR), which are self-explanatory. Sometimes, the term Allow Natural Death (AND) is used instead of DNI or DNR. If the patient is not admitted, one can discuss the option of "Do not hospitalize" or "Do not transfer to ICU". The key to making these decisions remains good communication, and then documentation of that communication. Ensuring comfort requires that specific measures are taken. Controlling pain then becomes the top priority. This pain may be from the disease, from artificial indwelling devices like the endotracheal tube, from immobility, from a distended bladder or bowel and each of these needs to be identified and controlled. Opiates are usually the first line option for relief of most pain, but other modalities should be used as liberally as needed. Dyspnea is an extremely unpleasant sensation, and the appropriate use of opiates and non-invasive ventilation (NIV) (if patient is not intubated) can relieve the distress. Both should be used as liberally as is necessary to ensure comfort. Retained secretions in the mouth or airway, drooling of these secretions can cause distress and repeated suction relieves this. Equally important is to ensure dignity and family access. There is little or no role of limiting visitors in the terminal phase. As long as other patients are not disturbed, the visitors' access should be as liberal as the patient or family want. Another important aspect of quality of life and preventing distress is to ensure that patients' autonomy is not overridden. Absence of control causes a sense of helplessness. Constantly communicating with the patients and seeking input and agreement into each therapeutic act avoids this. It is important the doctors continue to guide patients through these decisions, but one should ensure that the patient is involved in the process. Clearing decisions with family and not involving the patient directly only increases the loss of control and autonomy that the patient feels.

A recent large multinational study across Asia[1] looked at physician attitudes towards WH and WD treatment at EoL. Striking differences between Asian countries and the developed nations were present with regards to WH or WD treatment. An example used was a patient with hypoxic-ischemic encephalopathy with shock. In Asia, 53.8% were likely to continue do everything possible for said patient while <40% would in the USA and <10% would in Australia and some parts of Europe. Even implementation of DNR orders was significantly different among the various Asian countries with China, Bangladesh and Taiwan much less likely to implement them. Over half of physicians surveyed, 56.1%, would be reluctant to have limitation of treatment discussions with families. Religion, socio-economic status and a fear of litigation all seemed to play a role in the physicians' decision making. In view of the variability of perceptions across Asia, this study also highlighted the need for EoL care to be tailored to the needs of the region and country.

Indian Scenario

The Indian scenario is blighted by a legal vacuum. End of Life in ICU did not really exist when the constitution was drafted. Since then, there have been no laws or major judgement passed regarding the legality of EoL care specifically in ICU. Different medical and legal authorities have taken differing interpretations of the law. There have been a series of Indian papers published describing EoL in ICUs. These are usually from academic or tertiary institutes and may not reflect other ground level reality.[2-4] The Indian Society of Critical Care Medicine (ISCCM) framed a position statement and subsequently guidelines and later still an integrated care plan.[5-7]

There have been two Law Commissioners reports in the last decade. The Law Commissioner is the legal officer of the parliament and part of their role is to write the new draft laws for parliament which is then debated. If the draft laws get accepted, it becomes law. On two occasions, the law commissioner has drafted laws specifically related to EoL care in India, one in 2006 and the other in 2012. As of now neither has been reviewed and passed by parliament, so neither are law.

The first was the 196th Law Commission Report by Justice Jagannadha Rao in 2006. The main points from an ICU perspective are:

- Emphasizes the difference between Withdrawal Of Life Support (WOLS) and "euthanasia or assisted suicide"
- Legalizes WOLS where appropriate
- Provides protection for doctors performing appropriate EoL decisions
- Focuses on minimizing abuse of the law
- Acknowledges ISCCM's role
- BUT does not recognize patient autonomy or the living will

As there is no law that addresses specifics of EoL care in medical settings in India, the Aruna Shanbag judgement stands as law.

In the UK, Scenario 2a could occasionally happen.

The second was the 241st Law Commission report Justice PV Reddi (2012), who stated "Passive euthanasia", which is allowed in many countries, shall have legal recognition in our country too, subject to certain safeguards, as suggested by the 196th report and as held by the Supreme Court in *Aruna's case [(2011) 4 SCC 454)].It is not objectionable from legal and constitutional point of view."*

The constitution recognizes general right to life, and self determination. Euthanasia and suicide are currently illegal. As there is no law which addresses specifics of EoL care in medical settings in India, the most recent judgement stands as law. Currently, this is the Aruna Shanbag case and extracts of the judgement are reproduced verbatim below (Appendix 1). The reader can make up his or her own mind as to whether EoL limitation of care is legal or not in India.

UK Perspective

Of the two scenarios discussed earlier, in the UK, Scenario 2a could occasionally happen but Scenario 2b is unthinkable. Discussed below is EoL care for National Health Service (NHS) hospitals.

In the UK, the Liverpool End of Life Care pathway (LCP), a hospice style pathway for use in the hospital setting, was followed for managing end of life care. When the pathway was used well it did significantly lessen suffering at the EoL but following concerns raised and an independent review in 2013 the LCP was phased out in 2014. Priorities for care, which sets out 5 individualized priorities, replaced the LCP in July 2014.

The LCP was developed by the Royal Liverpool and Broadgreen University Hospitals NHS Trust hospital palliative care team and the Marie Curie Hospice in Liverpool in the 1990s. Although, this pathway was originally developed in Liverpool for the care of terminally ill cancer patients, it was implemented across the NHS (except in Wales). The reason for the design and implementation was the patchy delivery of EoL care across all healthcare systems although hospices did provide excellent EoL care and were considered a model of excellence in this respect. The LCP was adapted to a hospital setting to ensure patients received a high standard of care in the last hours and days of their life thus leading to a dignified and peaceful end to life and was designed for use during the last 72 hours of life once a diagnosis of "dying" was clearly established. In its nearly 20 year history, the LCP was considered as a model for best practice in EoL care and continued to get a clean bill of health from various national organizations as well as the Royal Colleges. The LCP then made its way into the specialist arena and specifically into critical care, a specialty where the emphasis is on saving lives and the focus on reducing mortality and improving quality of life. So, how did the two marry up especially as most patients on intensive care are unable to have their wishes known and rely heavily on surrogates to fill this gap.

One of the few common things about Critical care and palliative care are the number of patients at EoL that each specialty witnesses and has to deal with. One of the differences though is that patients and their families that are under palliative care teams have time to prepare for the eventuality of dying. The same unfortunately does not apply to intensive care. The LCP which was a generic version evolved from version 1 to version 12. Version 12 was modified into the speciality LCP ICU Model Pathway. This was around 2009 and was first implemented in Liverpool and then slowly made its way in some shape or form to other intensive care units in the country. This was based on the core principles that centered around assessment, communication and symptom management. It still didn't take away from the fact that, on an intensive care unit it is inherently difficult to diagnose a patient at EoL, thanks to the technology and the need to continue active treatment. But once the diagnosis was made it helped staff deliver holistic care.

Unfortunately, the LCP in Intensive Care had a very short life span. How then, did all of this come to an abrupt end?

The LCP that was supposed to provide guidance, to those not dealing with EoL care regularly, with a framework in how to care for patients at EoL. It slowly metamorphosed from being a guideline that could be individualized, to becoming a protocol to be rigidly followed, sometimes inappropriately. In some ways, it became a tick box exercise and where most clinicians would have documented that the patient was dying in the notes, the language over time changed to 'this patient fits the criteria for LCP', something that families failed to understand and the clinicians failed to explain. This led to media hype about the inappropriateness of the LCP and the associated issues around incentive payments made by the government to encourage the use of the pathway to improve care helped fuel the fire.

Transferring a ventilated end of life patient home to be extubated there, would be unthinkable in the UK.

Given that 19000 patients die every year on intensive care in the UK alone, managing EoL care is imperative.

One of the criticisms of the LCP was its name, a pathway, but not a pathway to recovery but rather a pathway to death, a concept that few were able to digest. Another was the perception that it hastened death.

This then led to the review headed by Baroness Julia Neuberger[8] which in effect criticized the lack of evidence to support the use of the LCP, an issue that would have been impossible to resolve as its near impossible to design a randomized controlled trial in dying patients with quality of death as an endpoint. Similarly, the review panel did not provide any evidence to suggest that it was the pathway, as a tool, which was at fault. Although, this review did mention some examples of excellent care when the pathway was appropriately used, it did not suggest any improvements to the LCP but instead wrote its death warrant and recommended an "End of life care plan".

So where are we now?

Mortality on UK intensive care units is approximately 15% with a hospital mortality of 22%,[9] that's nearly 19000 patients dying every year in intensive care. It is therefore imperative that EoL care is managed well as there is only one chance to get it right. While the LCP no longer exists, the void has been filled with the NICE Quality Standard for End of Life Care for adults (2011), a compilation of 16 quality standards that include identification, assessment, accessibility and consistent delivery of holistic care, and the document 'One Chance to Get it Right' by the Leadership Alliance for the Care of Dying People. In addition, the GMC guidance published in 2010 provides doctors with a framework to work towards ensuring appropriate care at the EoL for patients.

Legal Stance: In the UK, the principle of "best interest" is the fundamental principle that governs what medical treatment patients who lack capacity receive. The Mental Capacity Act of 2005 provides the legal framework as set by the UK Parliament for patients that lack capacity to make their own decisions. It clearly states: *Where the determination relates to life - sustaining treatment he (the person making the decision) must not, in considering whether the treatment is in the best interests of the person concerned, be motivated by a desire to bring about his death.*

Another concept that is enshrined in law is respect for autonomy and this applies to patients with capacity. Therefore, Advance Directives and Advance refusals for treatment are also binding.[10] Thus, competent patients have the right to refuse treatment but as per UK law do not have the right to demand certain treatments.

The focus on intensive care is firstly decision making around limiting, WH and WD treatment and secondly communicating with the families and next of kin of the patient and ensuring that everyone understands and is in agreement with the medical plan. Religious beliefs of the patient should also be ascertained and if requested by the family, chaplaincy services should be contacted. Most ICUs have protocols in place to guide the care once these decisions have been made. The focus of the protocols for limitation of treatment must center around precise instructions rather than ambiguous statements and must be clearly documented in the notes. The same applies to WH treatment. With WD of treatment consideration should be given to the family members and their wishes before the process is commenced. Another thing to consider is Organ Donation, especially when the decision is to WD treatment. On ICU as most patients are unable to voice their wishes it is imperative to check with the family members regarding any specific views the patient may have had or expressed during their life regarding organ and tissue donation. Advice can also be sought from the Local Transplant Coordinator which every ICU in the NHS has access to.

Brain Stem Death

A special mention is needed for brain stem death. Given the mortality on ICU, it is inevitable that clinicians are required to diagnose and confirm death. Death is defined as an irreversible cessation of consciousness combined with an irreversible cessation of respiration.[11] Death by cardiovascular criteria is relatively easy to diagnose. The clinician needs to confirm the irreversible cessation of pupillary, cardiac and respiratory activity. On the other hand Death by Neurological criteria can prove to be tricky for the uninitiated.

In India, the diagnosis of brain death falls under the organ transplant act. If there is consent for organ donation, the situation is straightforward. The brain death tests are done twice by two physicians and the patient/body is sent to the operation theatre for organ retrieval. This can only be done by designated physicians in institutes recognized by the zonal transplant

Diagnosing death by neurological criteria can be tricky for the uninitiated.

Clinicians need to be truthful and transparent about the terminal nature of the disease. All efforts must be made to ensure comfort and absence of suffering.

authorities. If the family is not willing for organ donation, the situation is less clear. One opinion is that death has occurred, regardless, and the patient/body can be disconnected from the ventilator and after the heart stops, the body can be handed over to the relatives. Another opinion is that this procedure is not legally valid as the brain death act is only pertinent in the context of organ donation for transplantation. In such a situation, especially where the relatives are unable to comprehend the meaning of brain death, it is best to ensure that every decision is preceded by extensive communication and documentation. If there is a wide consensus that further management is meaningless, and this is documented, the patient/body can be disconnected from the ventilator. Currently, it is still customary to document the time of death when the heart stops, rather than when the second set of tests were completed and brain death declared.

In the UK, there is no statutory definition of death. It was in 1976 following a proposal by the Conference of Medical Royal Colleges regarding "brain death criteria" that the UK courts adopted these criteria as part of law for the diagnosis of death.[11] To diagnose a patient as being brain stem dead requires strict adherence to guidelines for confirmation of death which include irreversible brain damage of known etiology, absence of brain stem reflexes and complete cessation of spontaneous respiration. It requires two medical practitioners who are registered for a minimum of 5 years to perform two sets of tests in order to confirm brain stem death. There is no prescribed interval between tests but death cannot be confirmed till both sets of tests are performed although the legal time of death is the time the first set of tests confirmed absence of brain stem reflexes.[11,12]

Conclusion

In summary, all the clinicians' first need to be is truthful and transparent about the prognosis and the potential terminal nature of the disease. Then the various options for limitation of care need to be discussed. Regardless of the degree of limitation, all efforts must be made to ensure comfort and absence of suffering. At end of life its important that patient dignity is maintained at all times.

Appendix 1

The judgement was delivered by Markandey Katju, J.

The arguments for allowing limitation of care were argued by Mr. Andhyarujina as the *amicus curiae* (friend of the court)

The arguments against allowing limitation of care were argued by Mr. Shekhar Naphade the learned Attorney General

Selected relevant abstracts are reproduced below:

IN THE SUPREME COURT OF INDIA CRIMINAL ORIGINAL JURISDICTION

WRIT PETITION (CRIMINAL) NO. 115 OF 2009

Aruna Ramchandra Shanbaug versus- Union of India and others

J U D G M E N T: Markandey Katju, J.

2. Euthanasia is one of the most perplexing issues which the courts and legislatures all over the world are facing today. This Court, in this case, is facing the same issue, and we feel like a ship in an uncharted sea, seeking some guidance by the light thrown by the legislations and judicial pronouncements of foreign countries, as well as the submissions of learned counsels before us. (Page 2)

4. We could have dismissed this petition on the short ground that under Article 32 of the Constitution of India (unlike Article 226) the petitioner has to prove violation of a fundamental right, and it has been held by the Constitution Bench decision of this Court in **Gian Kaur vs. State of Punjab**, 1996(2) SCC 648 (vide paragraphs 22 and 23) that the right to life guaranteed by Article 21 of the Constitution does not include the right to die. Hence, the petitioner has not shown violation of any of her fundamental rights. However, in view of the importance of the issues involved we decided to go deeper into the merits of the case. (Page 4)

Learned Attorney General stated that the report of the Law Commission of India on euthanasia has not been accepted by the Government of India. He further submitted that Indian society is emotional and care-oriented. We do not send our parents to old age homes, as happens in

Euthanasia is one of the most perplexing issues which the courts and legislatures all over the world are facing today.

The patient possesses the right not to consent i.e. to refuse treatment. This is known as the principle of self-determination or informed consent.

the West. He stated that there was a great danger in permitting euthanasia that the relatives of a person may conspire with doctors and get him killed to inherit his property. He further submitted that tomorrow there may be a cure to a medical state perceived as incurable today.

22. Mr. T. R. Andhyarujina, learned senior counsel whom we had appointed as Amicus Curiae, in his erudite submissions explained to us the law on the point. He submitted that in general in common law it is the right of every individual to have the control of his own person free from all restraints or interferences of others. Every human being of adult years and sound mind has a right to determine what shall be done with his own body. In the case of medical treatment, for example, a surgeon who performs an operation without the patient's consent commits assault or battery.

23. It follows as a corollary that the patient possesses the right not to consent i.e. to refuse treatment. (In the United States this right is reinforced by a Constitutional right of privacy). This is known as the principle of self-determination or informed consent.

24. Mr. Andhyarujina submitted that the principle of self-determination applies when a patient of sound mind requires that life support should be discontinued. The same principle applies where a patient's consent has been expressed at an earlier date before he became unconscious or otherwise incapable of communicating it as by a 'living will' or by giving written authority to doctors in anticipation of his incompetent situation.

Mr. Andhyarujina differed from the view of the learned Attorney General in that while the latter opposed even passive euthanasia, Mr. Andhyarujina was in favour of passive euthanasia provided the decision to discontinue life support was taken by responsible medical practitioners. (pages 34-35)

25. **If the doctor acts on such consent there is no question of the patient committing suicide or of the doctor having aided or abetted him in doing so.** It is simply that the patient, as he is entitled to do, declines to consent to treatment which might or would have the effect of prolonging his life and the doctor has in accordance with his duties complied with the patient's wishes. (Page 36)

26. The troublesome question is what happens when the patient is in no condition to be able to say whether or not he consents to discontinuance of the treatment and has also given no prior indication of his wishes with regard to it as in the case of Aruna. ....(Page 36)

27. Absent any indication from a patient who is incompetent the test which is adopted by Courts is what is in the best interest of the patient whose life is artificially prolonged by such life support. This is not a question whether it is in the best interest of the patient that he should die. The question is whether it is in the best interest of the patient that his life should be prolonged by the continuance of the life support treatment. This opinion must be formed by a responsible and competent body of medical persons in charge of the patient. (Page 37)

- **WITHDRAWAL OF LIFE SUPPORT OF A PATIENT IN PERMANENT VEGETATIVE STATE (PVS)**

126. There is no statutory provision in our country as to the legal procedure for withdrawing life support to a person in PVS or who is otherwise incompetent to take a decision in this connection. **We agree with Mr. Andhyarujina (*amicus curiae*) that passive euthanasia should be permitted in our country in certain situations, and we disagree with the learned Attorney General (Mr. Shekhar Naphade) that it should never be permitted.** (Pages 98-99)

References

1. Phua J, Joynt GM, Nishimura M, *et al.* Withholding and withdrawal of life-sustaining treatments in intensive care units in Asia. *JAMA Intern Med* 2015;175(3):363-71.
2. Kapadia F, Singh M, Divatia J, *et al.* Limitation and withdrawal of intensive therapy at end of life: practices in intensive care units in Mumbai, India. *Crit Care Med* 2005; 33:1272–75.
3. Mani RK, Mandal AK, Bal S, *et al.* End-of-life decisions in an Indian intensive care unit. *Intensive Care Med* 2009;35:1713–9.
4. Barnett VT, Aurora VK. Physician beliefs and practices regarding end of life care in India. *Indian J Crit Care Med* 2008;12:109–15.
5. Myatra SN, Salins N, Iyer S, *et al.* End-of-life care policy: An integrated care plan for the dying. *Indian J Crit Care Med* 2014;18:615–35.
6. Mani R K, Amin P, Chawla R, *et al.* Guidelines for end-of-life and palliative care in Indian intensive care units: ISCCM consensus Ethical Position Statement. *Indian J Crit Care Med* 2012;16:166–81.
7. Mani RK, Amin P, Chawla R, *et al.* Limiting life-prolonging interventions and providing palliative care towards the end-of-life in Indian intensive care units. *Indian J Crit Care Med* 2005;9:96–107.
8. More care less pathway: a review of the Liverpool Care Pathway. https://www.gov.uk/government/publications/reviewof-liverpool-care-pathway-for-dying-patients.
9. ICNARC: Key statistics from the Case Mix Programme 2012/2013.
10. The Mental Capacity Act 2005: Chapter 9, Part 1: 4 (5).
11. Academy of the Medical Royal Colleges. A Code of Practice for the Diagnosis and Confirmation of Death. London, 2008. Available from www.aomrc.org.uk/reports.aspx
12. Intensive Care Society (2005) Guidelines for Adult Organ and Tissue Donation. www.ics.ac.uk.

Summary of Pitfalls

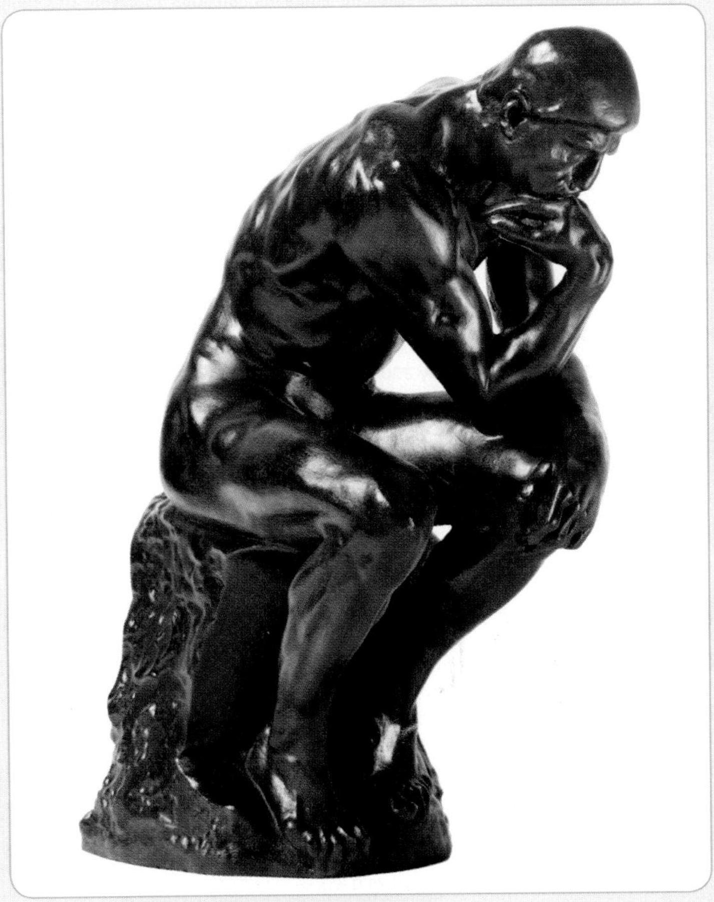

Summary of Pitfalls

Intensivists routinely deal with life threatening illnesses, anxious relatives and multiple colleagues from other specialties. The intensive care services consist of consultants, residents or trainees, nurses, and occasionally respiratory therapists. These ICU personnel have to communicate incessantly with each other and with other departments such as the Emergency Department, the Operation Theaters, the Imaging Services, the Laboratory Staff and the Blood Bank. At every step of the way, there is a potential for delay or worse error. Many of these can be costly in terms of worsening clinical outcomes. In this maze of conflicting demands, it is important for the ICU to deliver a smooth and efficient service. The two primary goals are to keep the patient alive and rapidly identify and reverse the triggering illness. The third role of the intensivist is to create an infrastructure than ensures that the above two are delivered rapidly and efficiently. Obviously ICU personnel need to be appropriately trained, up to date with current concepts and literature, but this alone is not enough. The delivery of care too must be seamless.

There are many reasons why this efficient care may not reach the patient and we feel that avoiding the 10 pitfalls below will result in better patient outcomes.

Pitfall No. 1: Delay in giving antibiotics in Septic Shock

Delay in rapid reversal of disease and resuscitation in other emergencies.

It is vital to ensure that reversal of the etiology of the disease is done as rapidly as possible. As illustrated in the case scenario, it is not uncommon to find that the need to resuscitate and stabilize the patient results in delay of definitive therapy. As in this scenario, delay in administering antibiotics can be associated with worse clinical outcomes.

Pitfall No. 2: Poor Hand washing and Infection control Practices

Infection control is one of the greatest, if not the single greatest achievement of medicine in the last 2-3 centuries. Intensive Care Unit patients are vulnerable and can get infected by cross contamination with ICU organisms and also with their own endogenous bacteria. Strict infection control practices focused on sterility at the point of contact with the patient and with indwelling devices will limit exogenous infections. Rapid reversal of primary illness and resuscitation will allow quick recovery and limit the potential for endogenous infections. Clear protocols and policies help in implementing these infection control practices.

Pitfall No. 3: Following Eminence Based rather than Evidence Based Medicine for basic ICU therapies

Intensivists and clinicians need to be updated with the important trials for the standard ICU techniques used to keep a patient alive. There have been a large number of trials in the last decade covering the best way to achieve hemodynamic stabilization, use mechanical ventilation and renal replacement therapy. There are still a large amount of unanswered questions regarding the use of these therapies.

Summary of evidence for CVS-RS-Renal support in the critically ill patient.

Hemodynamic

BP Target

- When following a pressure target, ensure that perfusion is maintained at that target.
- In septic shock target MBP of >65 mmHg, except in previously hypertensive patients in whom target >80–85 mmHg.
- Intra-operatively, prevent even brief periods of hypotension by avoiding MBP of less than 55 mmHg.
- In exsanguinating trauma accept low SBP of 70 or MBP of 50 mmHg till the bleeding has been surgically controlled.

Choice of Fluids for resuscitation

- In general crystalloids and colloids are associated with similar outcomes.
- The use of starch solutions may be deleterious in patients with renal injury or with the more severe forms of sepsis and they should be avoided in these patients.

- Routine replacement of albumin is not useful, but some sub group analysis and a meta-analysis suggest that it might be beneficial in severe sepsis.

Choice of vasoactive drug for shock

- Catecholamines seem equivalent for major outcomes.
- Safety profile and efficacy of Noradrenaline may be best overall and in cardiac patients.
- Vasopressin in low fixed dose a safe and effective alternative.

Ventilation

ARDS

- Use low TV and PAP as a default setting.
- In severe ARDS, high PEEP may be advantageous.
- Prone position ventilation is beneficial in severe ARDS.
- Techniques for reversing critical hypoxemia like NO or RM should only be used as rescue techniques and not as routine part of management.
- Alternatives like HFOV and ECMO need further evaluation to identify how best to use them. Currently their use should be limited to centers with enough experience and expertise, or in the context of patients being part of an RCT further evaluating these techniques.

Weaning

- Weaning using PSV or T-piece is preferable to SIMV.
- Use of protocols speeds up the weaning process.

NIV

- There is strong evidence of efficacy in acute exacerbation of COPD, acute cardiogenic pulmonary edema, immune compromised and in facilitation from weaning in COPD.
- There is intermediate evidence of efficacy in asthma, COPD with CAP, hypoxemic respiratory failure, post operative respiratory failure and in DNI-DNR patients.

Tracheostomy

- Routine early tracheostomy in those estimated to require prolonged ventilation is not justified based on the present evidence.

Renal

- Renal dose dopamine is ineffective and should not be used.
- Diuretics should be used to limit oliguria and fluid overload.
- HD and CRRT appear to have similar clinical outcomes.
- Standard intensity and high intensity RRT appear to have similar outcomes.
- The timing of initiation of RRT is unclear.

Pitfall No. 4: Wrong Therapeutic target

It is important to maintain focus on clinical outcomes rather than surrogate ones. It is relatively easy to target and monitor physiology and presume that this is improving clinical outcomes, but this is often not the case. Clinicians must be aware of the literature which demonstrates which physiological targets result in better clinical outcomes and which ones do not. One could then limit therapy to those that improve both surrogate and clinical outcomes.

Pitfall No. 5: Doing too much. Can Less be More?

The list of routine yet unproven therapies used in ICU appears endless. We have presented the evidence behind many of our standard therapies and noted that the majority of trials have failed to demonstrate patient benefit. Many have shown harm. In this context, it appears intuitive to be restrictive rather than liberal when selecting therapies for the critically ill in ICU. As an additional benefit, being restrictive will also prevent waste of resources, and in today's world, this equally applies to the rich and poor parts of the world.

Pitfall No. 6: Inadequate or inappropriate use of protocols and guidelines

A 3 fold approach to protocols and guidelines will help both, to prevent disasters and to promote excellence.

- Obsessively follow pragmatic protocols to enhance safety.
- Largely follow other guidelines based on high quality evidence.
- Resist slavishly following other guidelines based on poor quality evidence.

Pitfall No. 7: Inadequate communication and documentation

Communication and documentation in ICU is multifaceted. This includes communication within members of the ICU team and with personnel from other departments in the hospital. Communication between the patient or relatives and caregivers should be ensured, and lastly, free access for relatives to visit the patient further improves communication as well as reassures the patient

Pitfall No. 8: Inadequate Staffing

Intensive Care Units require a high number of trained staff. Critically ill patients on life support usually require 1:1 nursing ratio and occasionally even more, while a lower number is needed for those in ICU for observation, or for those in high dependency or step down units. Some ICUs also have respiratory therapists as part of the team. Adequate resident medical personnel are needed, to cover the ICU, to transport patients and to manage Rapid Response and Cardiac Arrest calls-and occasionally to help in the Emergency Department. Consultant should be in or immediately available to the ICU in daytime hours and contactable out of hours. Obviously, all ICU personnel should have appropriate levels of training.

Pitfall No. 9: Inadequate or delayed rehabilitation

Critical illness is followed by profound weakness and other organ system dysfunction. Physiotherapy and rehabilitation programs should be started as soon as possible during the critical illness and even when on mechanical ventilation rather than after ICU and hospital discharge.

Pitfall No. 10: Absence of EOL care planning

Firstly, all clinicians need to be truthful and transparent about the prognosis and the potential terminal nature of the disease. Then the various options for limitation of care need to be discussed. Regardless of the degree of limitation, all efforts must be made to ensure comfort and absence of suffering. At end of life it's important that patient dignity is maintained at all times.

Conclusion

We would like to conclude by noting that the foundation of modern intensive care is sound science, and would like to quote excerpts of a talk by Richard Feynman (emphasis by authors)

on what is and what is not science, how integrity to the scientific process is the foundation of good science and how external forces can compromise that integrity.

Cargo Cult Science Richard Feynman.

Some Remarks on Science, Pseudoscience, and Learning on How to Not Fool Yourself

The 1974 Caltech Commencement Address

In the South Seas, there is a cargo cult of people. During the war, they saw airplanes with lots of good materials, and they want the same thing to happen now. So they've arranged to make things such as runways, to put fires along the sides of the runways, to make a wooden hut for a man to sit in, with two wooden pieces on his head to headphones and bars of bamboo sticking out such as antennas--he's the controller--and they wait for the airplanes to land. They're doing everything right. The form is perfect. It looks exactly the way it looked before. But it doesn't work. No airplanes land. So I call these things cargo cult science, because they follow all the apparent precepts and forms of scientific investigation, but they're missing something essential, because the planes don't land.

Now it behooves me, of course, to tell you what they're missing. But it would be just about as difficult to explain to the South Sea islanders how they have to arrange things so that they get some wealth in their system. It is not something simple like telling them how to improve the shapes of the earphones. But there is one feature I notice that is generally missing in cargo cult science. That is the idea that we all hope you have learned in studying science in school--we never say explicitly what this is, but just hope that you catch on by all the examples of scientific investigation. *It is interesting, therefore, to bring it out now and speak of it explicitly. It's a kind of scientific integrity, a principle of scientific thought that corresponds to a kind of utter honesty--a kind of leaning over backwards*. For example, if you're doing an experiment, you should report everything that you think might make it invalid--not only what you think is right about it: other causes that could possibly explain your results; and things you thought of that you've eliminated by some other experiment, and how they worked--to make sure the other fellow can tell they have been eliminated.

Details that could throw doubt on your interpretation must be given, if you know them. You must do the best you can--if you know anything at all wrong, or possibly wrong--to explain it. If you make a theory, for example, and advertise it, or put it out, then you must also put down all the facts that disagree with it, as well as those that agree with it. There is also a more subtle problem. When you have put a lot of ideas together to make an elaborate theory, you want to make sure, when explaining what it fits, that those things it fits are not just the things that gave you the idea for the theory; but that the finished theory makes something else come out right, in addition.

In summary, the idea is to give all of the information to help others to judge the value of your contribution; not just the information that leads to judgment in one particular direction or another.

....

We've learned from experience that the truth will come out. Other experimenters will repeat your experiment and find out whether you were wrong or right. Nature's phenomena will agree or they'll disagree with your theory. And, although you may gain some temporary fame and excitement, you will not gain a good reputation as a scientist if you haven't tried to be very careful in this kind of work. *And it's this type of integrity, this kind of care not to fool yourself, that is missing to a large extent in much of the research in cargo cult science.*

....

It is very dangerous to have such a policy in teaching--to teach students only how to get certain results, rather than how to do an experiment with scientific integrity.

So, I have just one wish for you--the good luck to be somewhere, where you are free to maintain the kind of integrity I have described, and where you do not feel forced by a need to maintain your position in the organization, or financial support, or so on, to lose your integrity. May you have that freedom?

APPENDIX

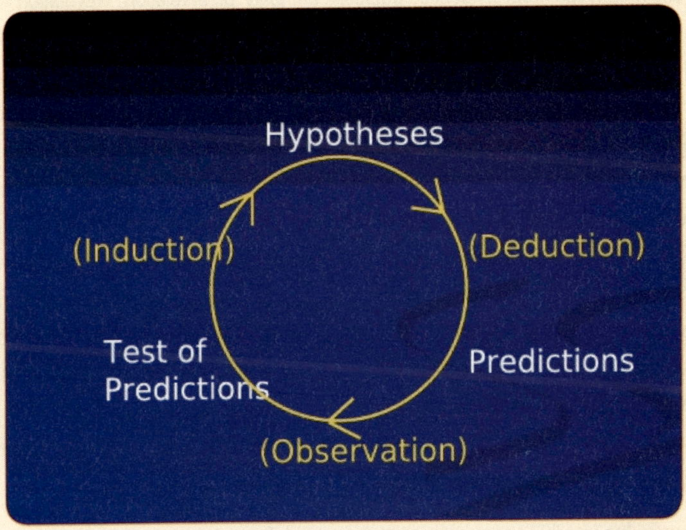

The Scientific Process

Appendix

A Practical Approach to Evidence Based Medicine (EBM)

We gain knowledge from evidence, tradition, authority or revelation. Revelation sounds quaint; someone has an intuition, believes it is a divine message, unquestionably accepts it and then expects others to blindly accept it too. Intuition is a way of obtaining knowledge, but it needs some sort of validation. Intuition is initially very useful, but beyond a point, is of limited value. Intuition is based on a series of mental projections and calculations, and the more numerous and complex the calculations, the more likely the intuited response will be fallacious. A simple example is to try and guess or intuit the numbers of different ways available for 10 people to sit on 10 chairs around a table. Very few people without a mathematical background will be close to the correct answer of greater than 3 million. Another example, called The Birthday Paradox, is often used to show how intuition can be misleading. The question is; what is the chance that at least 2 people on a football field share the same birthday. (Total of 23 people; 22 players and 1 referee). The correct answer is ~50% but most people will intuit a much lower figure. It is better to actually do the calculations than to rely on intuition. (See Figure 1 for explanation of above 2)

In science, the last 300 years have seen a major shift away from tradition and authority to empiricism and evidence. In this context, empiricism is best defined as "from experiment and observation". Eminence based medicine is a combination of tradition and authority and revelation. Clinical medicine too is shifting away from this unquestioning acceptance of the wisdom of tradition and authority. It is focused on framing plausible concepts, formulating testable hypotheses, designing experiments to test these ideas and seeing if the data matches the predictions. Some senior eminence based medicine practitioners have an interesting take on this whole evidence based medicine bandwagon. They claim their approach is based on wisdom, while others merely have knowledge. Regardless, it is worthwhile for all clinicians to have a working knowledge of the principles of EBM.

Correct answer for number of ways 10 people can sit on 10 chairs is 3,628,800 = 10!, or 10 factorial or 10 x 9 x 8 x 7 x 6 x 5x 4 x 3 x 2 x 1, as the first person has 10 chair options, the second has nine remaining chair options, the third has eight remaining chair options etc.

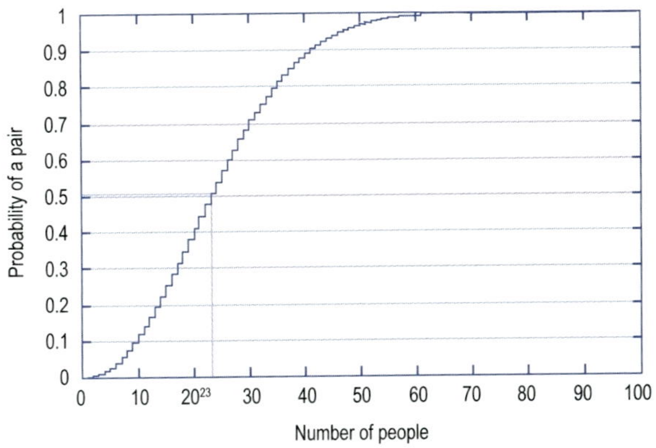

Figure 1:

Birthday Paradox: The graph shows the actual probability values for different numbers of people sharing a birthday.

Brief Explanation: It is easier to do the calculations by seeing the probability of all the people in the group not sharing a birthday. Then, the remaining is the probability of at least 2 people sharing a birthday. So, if there is a 90% probability of all the people in a group not sharing a birthday, it implies that there is a 10% chance of at least 2 people in that group sharing a birthday. The probability of 2 people not sharing a birthday is 365/365 x 364/365, as the first persons' birthday can be any of the 365 days of the year and the second has to be on any of the other 364 days. This means there is a 99.73% chance of 2 people not sharing a birthday. The chance of 3 people not sharing a birthday is 365/365 x 364/365 x 363/365 as the third persons' birthday has to be on any of the remaining 363 days. Now, the probability of these 3 people not sharing a birthday is 99.18%, a slightly lower probability than that of 2 people not sharing a birthday. Repeating, the probability of 4 people not sharing a birthday is 365/365 x 364/365 x 363/365 x 362/365 = 98.36%, the probability of 5 people not sharing is 365/365 x 364/365 x 363/365 x 362/365 x 361/365= 97.29%, etc. As the number of people included increase, the probability of all of them not sharing a birthday slowly decreases, as seen in the above series of calculations. When the number reaches 23, the probability of any of them not sharing a birthday reaches 49.3%, implying there is a 50.7% chance that at least two of the 23 people will share a birthday. (The above calculation is for a non leap-year and also makes the questionable presumption that birthdays occur randomly through the year).

Probably the greatest discovery in the history of knowledge and science was the "discovery of ignorance". This discovery forced people to sit back and try to figure out what really worked and what didn't. The whole scientific approach and process was an attempt to overcome the prevailing state of ignorance.

The figure at the beginning of this appendix shows this process.

Feynman encapsulated the essence of science in 1 minute of a talk. (The Essence of Science in 60 Seconds -Richard Feynman https://www.youtube.com/watch?v=5v8habYTfHU).

In general we look for a new law by the following process. First you guess. Don't laugh; this is the most important step. Then you compute the consequences.

Compare the consequences to experience / experiment. If it disagrees with experiment, then the guess is wrong. In that simple statement is the key to science.

It does not matter how beautiful your guess is or how smart you are or what your name is. If it disagrees with experience, it's wrong. That's all there is to it.

We can now apply these concepts directly to clinical trials.

To paraphrase Feynman in a medical context.

In general we look for a new law by the following process. In medicine, we are looking for a therapy, say albumin in septic shock.

First you guess. Don't laugh; this is the most important step. The concept that albumin is important is based on physiological knowledge, and the guess that it might be a better resuscitation fluid than saline because it will not leak from the circulation. This guess is based on the physiology that albumin will exert an oncotic pressure. As per Starlings forces, this oncotic pressure from inside the vessel will "pull" fluid into the circulation. Saline does not have a matching oncotic pressure, so the Starling forces will result in more water leaving the circulation. Also smaller studies earlier showed some benefits compared to saline. When we put all this together, it appears plausible and therefore sensible to study it in more detail.

Then you compute the consequences. If our guess were right, we would expect that patients receiving albumin would have faster resolution of hypotension and less edema. This would in turn lead to less renal dysfunction, less pulmonary edema, and subsequently less vasoactive medication, mechanical ventilation, renal replacement therapy and finally this would translate to lower mortality.

Compare the consequences to experience/experiment. Do an RCT in which half the septic shock patients are randomized to receive saline, the others to albumin as the resuscitation fluid. Document time to reverse hypotension, need for vasopressors, renal parameters, ventilator requirements, RRT requirements and mortality.

If it disagrees with experiment, then the guess is wrong. If the incidence of the above parameters are similar in both groups, we can conclude that our guess that albumin was a better resuscitation fluid than saline was wrong.

In that simple statement is the key to science. It does not matter how beautiful your guess is or how smart you are or what your name is. If it disagrees with experience, it's wrong. That's all there is to it. No amount of eminence and argument that one has seen patients get better with albumin is now going to change the fact that albumin did not turn out to be a superior resuscitation fluid to saline.

There is one ambiguous line in this passage... *If it disagrees with experiment*...Disagreement could mean anything. If the mortality with saline was 20% and with albumin was 19%, do we conclude that the result was positive or that it was negative? To answer this, we need to have a more detailed look at the concept of proof.

The Concept of Proof

"Science never proves anything. It offers various levels of disproof."

Before we proceed, we should look at the concept of randomness and the problem of large numbers.

The concept of Randomness: It is useful to define randomness here. It is a surprisingly recent concept. It was always assumed that everything occurred for a reason that could be the will of god, or a predestined fate, or the desire of the king. Gerolamo Cardano (1501-76) an Italian mathematician and gambler wrote a treatise "*The Book on Games of Chance*" in which he stated *"If a random event has several equally likely outcomes, the chance of any individual outcome occurring is equal to the proportion of that outcome to all possible outcomes"*. This means that the chance of a dice falling on the number 4 is exactly 1/6, as there are 6 possible ways it can fall. Or that the chance of picking any specific card from a deck, be it the mighty Ace of Spades or the lowly 3 of Hearts, is exactly 1/52 (1/54 if the Jokers are included). This seemingly obvious concept was so far ahead of its time that it was published one century after his death. Even today many people fail to grasp how much chance and randomness dictates events.

The Problem of Large Numbers explains why we need statistics. Two examples are often used to highlight "the problem of large numbers". The first is the story of the Indian king who offered one of his subjects, a mathematician, and a reward of his choice. The subject requested that one grain of rice be put on the 1st square of a chess board, double be put on the second square, double that on the third, etc. he requested that his reward be the grains of rice on the 64th or last square. The king granted what he thought was a meager reward, but when the calculations were done the answer was 18,446,744,073,709,551,615, well beyond both the king's and the earth's resources. The other observation is that the number of possible positions of 32 chess pieces on a chessboard is 10^{123}. To keep that in context, there are estimated to be 10^{80} atoms in the universe and 10^{17} seconds since the beginning of time.

In a medical context, if we look at one outcome, say mortality, for a given therapy in a sample size of 5000 patients, the total possibilities will overwhelm our capacity to do the study. As a result we make a probability calculation and assume that this will apply to the majority of patients.

What is proof?

Historically, the concept of proof is attributed to Pythagoras the Greek mathematician. Pythagoras' theorem is one of the most famous examples in mathematics, but it is not the theorem that is relevant here. It is the fact that there was a scheme to demonstrate that the theorem was true. This process of showing something to be inevitably true was the first concept of proof. One need to clarify that proof is only for predicting future events, not for past events. The aim of the scientific process is to overcome ignorance. The way to overcome ignorance is to try to predict events before they happen and be prepared for them or exploit them to one's advantage. To be successful in predicting events one tries to find patterns of events that are reliably reproducible. The more reliably a pattern is reproduced, the more confident we can be that the same pattern will occur in the future. Proof is a way of stating how reliable our predictions will be. It is important to put this clearly in context. One does not need a scientific process to observe past events. One needs a scientific method to predict future events.

Pythagoras' Theorem states; in any right-angled triangle the area of the square on the hypotenuse is equal to the sum of the areas of the squares of the other two sides. Figure 2 below is one example of its proof. This is a 100% proof. There is no possible example in which the theorem does not hold true. This 100% proof is called mathematical proof. It has been true for 1000's of years and it will remain true for 1000's of years to come. It is also called theoretical proof as one can see that the theorem is true without actually doing any experiments or taking any measurements.

However, there are many real world circumstances where we will never get 100% or absolute certainty. Here, we opt for another form of relative proof, called scientific or statistical proof.

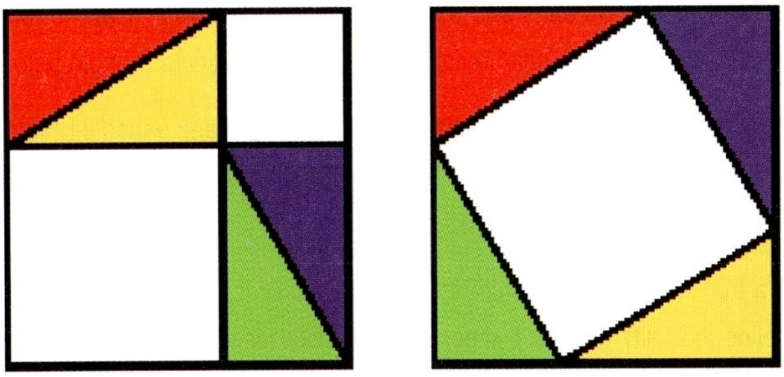

Figure 2. "BEHOLD" The proof of Pythogarus' Theorem

The exact origin if this particular example of proof of the theorem is unknown. It is believed to be of Chinese origin and also believed to have actually predated Pythagorean (570-459 BC) who framed the theorem. The great Indian mathematician, Bhaskara (1114-1118) found this proof so elegant, that he reproduced it in his book Lilavati without any explanation. Instead he simply titled it "Behold":

Scientific proof is sometimes called the poor relation of mathematical proof. Based on the calculated probability we can reach some tentative conclusions. For example, when we toss a coin, we assume that each toss has a 50% chance of falling heads or tails. This assumption is based on the fact that the coin actually has a heads and a tails, and it is equally weighted to fall with equal chance on either side. We then toss it say 10 times, and it falls on heads all 10 times. We can calculate the probability of this. Each toss has a 50% chance of heads. So for all 10 to fall on heads the probability would be $1/2^{10} = 1/1024$. This is such a small probability that it make us question our initial assumption that the probability of heads was actually 50%. Maybe this is a double head side coin, or a coin heavily weighted to fall towards heads. We make this assumption based on how rare the observation is, in this case 1/1024. If we tossed the coin 100 times and it fell on heads all 100 times, we would question our initial assumption more strongly.

We can do all the calculations for each observation and also show this numerically (Figure 3).

We first ask, how many ways we can get all 10 heads or all 10 tails. For each, there is only one way, all the tosses are heads or tails (1/1024). We then ask how many ways can we get 1 heads and 9 tails, the answer is 10/1024, as any one of the 10 tosses could be heads, as long as the other 9 fall on tails. Then, we ask how many ways can we get 2 heads, and the number will increase. So, there are many more combinations of the 1024 that will have 5 heads and 5 tails than have say, 2 heads and 8 tails. We can plot it as a graph below. At the left end is the 1/1024 probability of all heads and at the right end of all tails. Next comes 10 ways of getting 1 heads and 9 tails. Then comes 45 combinations of getting 2 heads and 8 tails, then 120 ways of getting 3 heads and 7 tails, 210 ways of getting 4 heads and 6 tails and 252 ways of getting 5 heads and 5 tails. Extending to 4, 3, 2, 1 and 0 tails, the total adds up to 1024. The numbers can be calculated by using Pascals' triangle below Figure 3.

They can now be put on a Bell or Gaussian Curve (Figure 4), and based on the observation we can check the P value. As the P value becomes smaller and smaller, it becomes less and less likely that the observation is a random event.

Similarly in a trial comparing 100 patients receiving albumin, to 100 receiving saline, with a known baseline mortality of 50% it is perfectly possible for all those receiving saline to die and all receiving albumin to survive, *purely as a random event*. It is just that the probability of this event is so low ($1/2^{200}$), that we reject it and say that albumin is advantageous compared to saline. Using such frequency statistics, one can calculate how common or rare a particular observation is, based purely on randomness or chance.

The calculated value of $1/2^{200}$ is the probability of all patients in one group dying and all in the other group surviving. It is called the "exact" probability as it is based purely on the study population.

1

1 1

1 2 1

1 3 3 1

1 4 6 4 1

1 5 10 10 5 1

1 6 15 20 15 6 1

1 7 21 35 35 21 7 1

1 8 28 56 70 56 28 8 1

1 9 36 84 126 126 84 36 9 1

1 10 45 120 210 252 210 120 45 10 1

All 10 Heads   5 Heads + 5 Tails   All 10 Tails

Figure 3. Pascals' Triangle: Each number is the sum of the two numbers above it. The number of rows is the number of events, in this case 10 tosses of the coin.

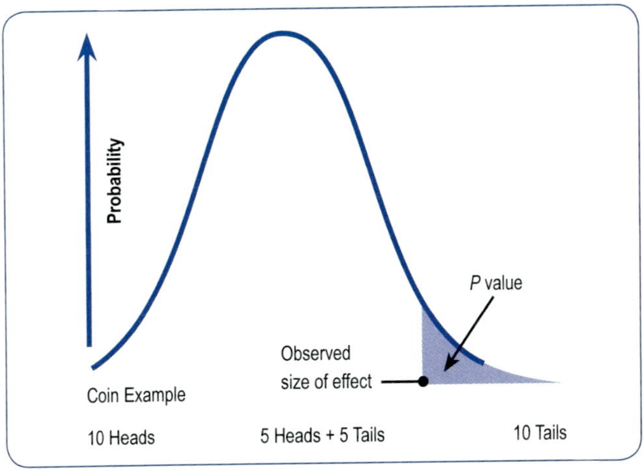

Figure 4. Gaussian Curve showing distribution of probabilities

The coin example had 2 outcomes, heads or tails. In clinical trials, we have 4 outcomes. For example, we could look at mortality in shock with the use of albumin or saline. The four outcomes are; received albumin and lived, received albumin and died, received saline and lived and received saline and died. We put this in a 2 x 2 table (Table 1). Unlike the coin example, where we know that there are only two possibilities of exactly 50%, heads or tails, in the clinical trial example, we can never be sure that the mortality will be an assured 50% (equal likelihood of survival or death). Also, in a clinical trial, we first take a smaller study sample from the larger population, then study that smaller representative population and subsequently apply our findings back in the larger overall patient population. We hope that our small study population actually represents the larger population of all patients with the disease. Because the mortality is not fixed, and it may be slightly different in the smaller study population compared to the overall general population, we do not go by the exact probability calculated in the study sample. Instead it is modified by the observed mortality. This P value is calculated from the 2 x 2 table (Table 1) using a test like the Chi squared test.

The choice of statistical analysis and test will depend on the kind of data being collected and studied, but the question is the same. Is this outcome so rare as to fall in the extreme 5% of probabilities?

It is apparent, that this will never be a 100% form of scientific or statistical proof, regardless of the number of observations. If a coin has fallen on heads 20 out of 20 times, we cannot with 100% certainty say that the next will also be heads. Similarly, if 100 of 100 patients receiving

Table 1. 2 x 2 Table. Hypothetical data in which there is a near equal mortality of ~ 50% in patients receiving either saline or albumin. In this example of 200 patients 110 got randomized to the albumin group.

	Albumin	Saline	Total
Lived	A = 50	B = 42	92
Died	C = 60	D = 48	108
Total	110	90	

saline die and 110 of 110 patients receiving albumin survive, we still cannot with 100% certainty say that the next patient to receive saline will die or the one to receive albumin will survive. In clinical medicine, we have to opt for a statistical or scientific probability based proof rather than a mathematical one purely because the number of probabilities is so high, that we cannot study them all, as discussed earlier in the problem of large numbers.

The example of the chessboard and domino (Figure 5) is often used to highlight the difference between theoretical or mathematical proof and scientific or statistical proof.

This picture represents a chessboard where the top left and bottom right white squares have been removed, leaving 62 squares. You have 31 dominos, each capable of exactly covering 2 squares. The question is, how many ways can you cover the 62 squares with these 31 dominos. The scientific approach would be to make a guess, say 1 in 20 patterns would cover all squares, then try 20 patterns and see if one can cover all 62 squares. If one cannot, one changes the guess to maybe 1 in 50 and repeats the experiment. And so on, till one finds the number than matches the guess. But in this case, no matter how many times one has tried, no pattern has covered all 62 squares. So the question now changes to; is it possible to cover all 62 squares with these 31 dominos. If one can test every possible pattern, we can answer the question, but the problem of large numbers appears. What if the total number of combinations of placing the 31 dominos is so large that one will not have time to test them all? The best one can say is that scientifically we have not found any pattern that will cover all 62 squares. We cannot be 100% certain about our conclusion till every possible combination has been tested.

The theoretical or mathematical proof will go as follows:

1. There are 64 - 2 = 62 squares
2. 32 are black and 30 are white
3. Pattern is alternate black and white. No 2 squares of the same color are adjacent

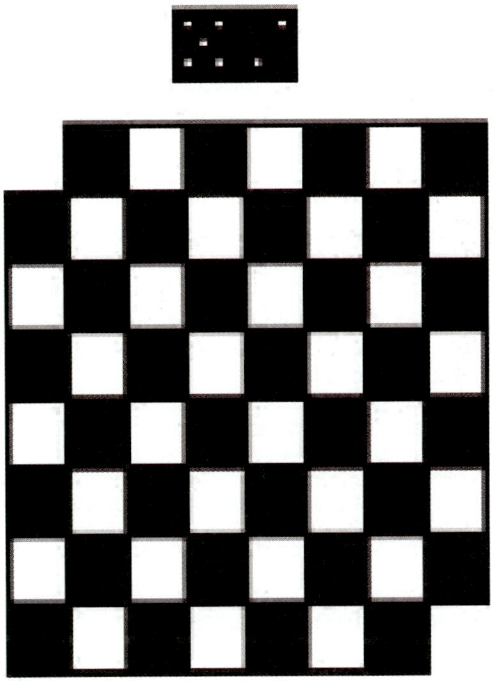

Figure 5. The Chess and Domino Problem

4. 30 dominos *in any possible combination* will cover 30 black and 30 white squares
5. Two non-adjacent black squares remain.
6. There is no way the 31st domino can cover these two non-adjacent black squares.

Conclusion: It is Impossible to cover all 62 squares with 31 dominos (100% or absolute proof). Without making a single measurement, one can reach a 100% conclusion, with no possible exception.

Conjecture and Theorem versus Hypothesis and Conclusion

As discussed initially, we first start with a guess, and if we can prove it, we believe it to be true. In Mathematics the guess is called a conjecture, and when proven, it becomes a theorem. In science, it is called a hypothesis, and when proven, it becomes a conclusion.

There are many examples in mathematics, where there is a conjecture that has not been formally proved, but it has never been shown to be wrong. In the case of mathematics, if even one example does not agree with the conjecture it is rejected as false. An example is a conjecture by the famous Swiss mathematician, Euler. He made a conjecture or claim that there were no solutions to the equation $x^4 + y^4 + z^4 = w^4$. Euler couldn't prove it. For the next 200 years no other mathematician could either prove it or find an example to disprove it, even when using the number crunching power of computers. So it was believed to be true, till in 1988 Elkies from Harvard gave this example:

$$2{,}682{,}440^4 + 15{,}365{,}639^4 + 18{,}796{,}760^4 = 20{,}615{,}673^4.$$

The conjecture was then rejected as false.

Scientific proof is not absolute, but it is good enough. A single exception does not make us reject a conclusion. If it is scientifically proven that noradrenaline increases the blood pressure, and we come across a patient in whom it does not increase the blood pressure, we do not reject noradrenaline as a useful drug in shock.

Statistics and Clinical Trials

When one uses the term scientifically proven, it is often assumed to be a 100% proof, when in reality it never is. It is only a degree of certainty. In medical science, the pragmatic two values that are considered as useful cutoffs are:

- $P < 0.05$ = Reliably Probable
- $P < 0.001$ = Exceedingly Probable

When we conduct a study, we compare two groups, one with treatment and one without the treatment. If the difference in outcome between the two groups is "statistically significant" we interpret it as the therapy is effective. We are guided by the *P* value in making this decision. A *P* value of <0.001 is more reliable than <0.05, but only in as much as it represents a more rare or extreme event under the assumption that the null hypothesis is correct.

Once we have decided that a therapy is effective, we than have to get an idea of how effective it is. We can do this in different ways. (We do *not* use the *P* value for this. The *P* value only tells us how common or rare the observation is). One way is to discuss the benefit in terms of risk reduction (RR). This may be in terms of relative RR (RRR) or absolute RR (ARR). Let's say a therapy decreases mortality from 40% in the placebo arm to 30% in the treatment arm. The ARR will be 40 - 30 = 10%. The relative risk will be 75% (as 30 is 75% of 40). So, the relative risk reduction will be 25% (100-75). Looking at these two numbers, *which are expressing exactly the same statistic;* it becomes obvious that one can opt to use

RRR to make the benefit appear larger. To prevent the reader from being misled, another option is to use Numbers Needed to Treat (NNT). This denotes how often a therapy must be used to save an additional life. It is calculated as 100/ARR. In this instance, the ARR will be 100/10 = 10. In the above example, if one treats 10 patients in each arm, there will be one additional life saved, as there will be 4/10 deaths in the placebo arm and 3/10 in the treatment arm. The lower the number, the more effective the treatment. As another example, a therapy decreases mortality from 0.3% in placebo arm to 0.1% in treatment arm. Here the ARR is 0.2% but the RRR is 66%. If only the RRR is given in the paper, the reader may be lead to believe the treatment is spectacularly successful, but if given the raw data, then it looks much less impressive. The NNT is 500 (100 / 0.2), that means after 500 people have received the treatment, one additional life is saved. It becomes apparent that this treatment is not that beneficial. The NNT is also a good way to judge how cost effective a treatment is. It obviously makes more sense to choose therapies with low NNTs, so more patients can benefit, and resources can be focused on therapies which benefit larger number of patients. It should be remembered that an NNT is specific to a time frame. The benefit of a treatment at 1 week may be different from that at 1 month, and the ARR and NNT will depend on the time point at which the data was collected.

Another way of looking at the data is to look at the RR and the 95% confidence interval (CI). In the first example above, the mortality is 30 and 40% so the RR is 0.75. (It could also be expressed as 1.3 if we flip the numerator and denominator i.e. we could express the ratio as 30:40 or as 40:30). Yet another way of expressing the benefit is the Odds Ratio (OR). To understand the difference between RR and OR one must understand the difference between calculating the Risk versus the Odds. In a sample of 100 patients of whom 30 die, the Risk of death is 30/100. The numerator is the number who died and the denominator is the total number of patients. The Odds of death are 30/70, the numerator is again the total number who died, but the denominator is the patients that survived. Thus, the RR is the ratio of the risk in the treatment arm versus that of the control arm and the OR is the ratio of the odds in the treatment arm vs. that of the control arm.

The CI is a way of expressing how reliable the RR or OR is. Before going to 95% CI it is worth understanding what the 100% CI is. Essentially it is a range in which one can be 100% certain that the correct value lies within that range. As an example, an opaque bag has hundred black or white balls. One is asked to guess the number of white balls, and a reasonable guess would be 50. One is then asked to give a range within which, with 100% certainty, the answer lies. The correct answer at this point is 0-100 as all or none of the balls may be white. Now one removes 10 balls and notes that 5 are white and 5 are black. Our guess would still be 50 balls are white, but the 100% CI now is 5-95 as we know that at least

5 balls are white, and since, there are at least 5 black balls, the maximum number of white balls can be 95. Then another 20 are removed, and 5 are white and 15 are black. Now the 100% CI has narrowed to 10-80. As the data on the number of balls increases, the 100% CI narrows.

The 95% CI is a variation in which we say that with 95% confidence we can say that the range of correct answers will be between these two limits.

To continue the above example, in this case we can say we guess that there are 50 white balls, and we can say with 95% certainty, that the range is 20-80 white balls.

Another way of looking at the 95% CI is to state that if we do a similar study a 100 times, the range will fall between these two limits at least 95 times. The narrower the confidence interval, the more reliable the result. In general, the larger the numbers studied, and the lower the standard deviation of the data, the narrower the confidence interval.

We use these basic statistic concepts to first decide if a treatment is effective, and then to decide how confident we can be about our result and finally to see the degree of efficacy of the treatment. There are many limitations and flaws to this approach that will be discussed later. Despite these limitations, these statistical concepts, used in large Randomized Clinical Trials (RCTs) and systematic reviews or meta-analysis are currently the most reliable way to evaluate treatments. In large double-blind randomized clinical trials we first ask a specific and focused question. We then estimate the frequency of the end point (e.g. expected mortality) and the expected benefit of the intervention. Based on this we then calculate a minimum number of patients needed. We screen patients to see if they fit our diagnosis and criteria, and if they do, we seek their consent. When they give consent, we randomize them, effectively deciding, with the toss of a coin, whether they get the treatment or the placebo. (Usually a computer does the randomization, but like the toss of a coin, the patient has an equal chance of ending up in either group). Once the consent is obtained and the patient is randomized, they are considered as enrolled in the study. The treatment is delivered in a way that neither the treating team, the investigating team nor the patients know if they are getting placebo or therapy. The patients are followed up, and all the relevant baseline data, and endpoint data is recorded. The advantage of randomizing and blinding is that there is minimal chance of bias, as it is difficult for either the patient or the investigators to influence the outcomes. Since many studies will be small, the results may not be reliable. A systematic review or meta-analysis is a way of combining many trials testing a similar treatment in a specific condition, combining the results, and hoping that the larger numbers analyzed will give a more statistically reliable answer.

Before we go into the details of reading papers there are two common errors readers should be aware of. Both will be explained with examples. In the first case, the flaw appears obvious and the resultant conclusion is absurd. The second pitfall, using the example with the medals, is less obvious. These two pitfalls are endemic in the medical literature and have lead many readers astray with erroneous conclusion. They largely contribute to the Cargo Cult Science of contemporary EBM.

The first pitfall concerns a study which was done in a hospital to evaluate their patient population, the practice patterns and outcomes. Data was collected for all patients in 1 year and this included ICU patients, In-Patients and Out-Patients. Data was collected regarding age, sex, ethnicity, admitting diagnosis, background diseases, surgical and interventional procedures done, medical treatment delivered, length of hospital stay and outcome (lived / died). The investigators got a useful idea about the kind of work the hospital does with this data. Later a statistician was asked to see if he could get any more information from the database. He made the following observations of hospital mortality that year. Intensive care unit mortality: 100/1000 (10%), In-Patient mortality: 100/10,000 (1%) and Out-Patient mortality: 1/1,00,000 (0.001%). He then did a P value calculation to see if this could be explained by chance, and found that the P value was highly significant between each of the groups. Based on this observation, he came to the conclusion that ICU was the worst place to get admitted to with a life threatening illness. Every clinician will recognize the absurdity of this conclusion, but most will not be able to pinpoint the fundamental flaw that lead to this absurd conclusion. The flaw is that this study was not designed to answer the question "where should one get admitted with a life threatening illness". Put another way, in this example, the methods and data collection *preceded* the hypothesis. In science, we first frame the question, and then design the study. This kind of error is widespread in literature and leads to a lot of confused conclusions. Data mining, finding a pattern, and then presenting it as a conclusion rather than a hypothesis that may be worth testing.

The second common pitfall is demonstrated in the medal table below (Figure 6). This was from the 2010 Delhi Commonwealth Games.

The question is, why did India come second and not England since; the latter had more medals totally. The answer is because India got more Gold medals. But one could argue that total medals should be given more importance that Gold medals. The real point is not whether Gold medals or total medals are more important. The point is that the decision has to be taken before the games start. If one could choose the system of ranking after the games are complete, one could choose a system that would favor one team over the other.

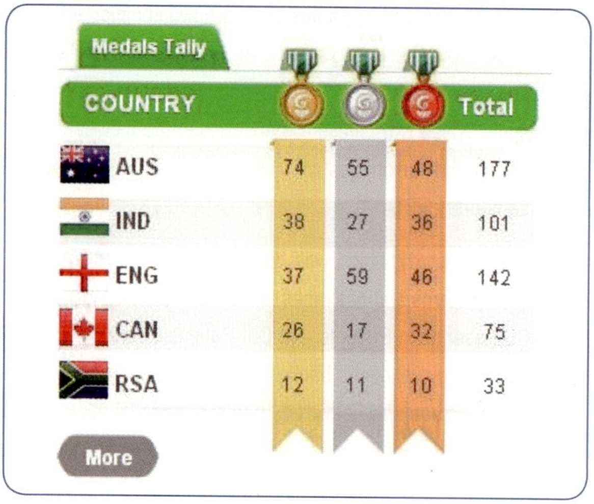
Medals Tally

COUNTRY	Gold	Silver	Bronze	Total
AUS	74	55	48	177
IND	38	27	36	101
ENG	37	59	46	142
CAN	26	17	32	75
RSA	12	11	10	33

More

Figure 6. Delhi Commonwealth Games 2010 Medal Table

This is called post hoc analysis. In many studies, the post hoc analysis is done, and then presented as a conclusion rather than a hypothesis that may be worth testing.

I now turn to another kind of principle or idea, and that is that there is no sense in calculating the probability or the chance that something happens after it happens. A lot of scientists don't even appreciate this........

– Richard Feynman: This Unscientific Age. The Danz Lectures: April 1963

Now moving on to RCTs and meta-analysis, a lot of which exist in literature. Below is a simplified scheme to read a RCT or a meta-analysis.

How to Read Randomized Clinical Trials or Meta-Analysis

This section is aimed for self-taught clinicians such as the authors who do not have a strong, or even a basic statistical grounding. It is necessarily simplified and brief, but we hope it gives an approach to get the most out of a paper. As an introduction, we suggest that the reader approaches the paper with an open mind, regardless of their current opinion on the subject. For example, if one is evaluating tight sugar control, and one believes it is beneficial, then, for the duration of reading the paper one should identify and suspend one's bias. The aim of reading the paper is to see what the data of that paper is telling you; in this case, maybe, does tight sugar control decrease 90 day mortality. The aim of reading the paper is not to simply confirm what one thinks is true. There is little point reading a paper if one will only accept the interpretation which confirms one's bias, and reject the conclusion if it does not agree with the reader's bias. All the examples in the below discussion have been covered in the earlier EBM chapters and the references will not be cited here again.

The CONSORT or Consolidated Standards of Reporting Trials guideline (http://www.consort-statement.org) for RCTs comprehensively reviews the subject.

Reading a Randomized Clinical Trial

Step 1: Understand the question or hypothesis in its entirety

Step 2: Check that the methods are appropriate and sound

Step 3: Go straight to the Tables and Figures

Step 4: Make your own initial interpretation

Step 5: Read the results and discussion in detail

Step 6: Make a final interpretation of the study

Step 1: Understand the question or hypothesis in it's entirety

When evaluating a hypothesis, one must clearly identify 4 components and the statistics (PICO+S)

- Patient
- Intervention
- Comparator
- Outcome (at specified time)

Each of this should be clearly defined in the introduction and methods section. For example, in the LaRS trial if the question was "do steroids work in ARDS?" this would not be a well framed hypothesis as there is too much ambiguity.

Looking at this question in terms of PICO+S

- Patient = those with ARDS as per the definition chosen.
- Intervention = late in ARDS (7-28 days) and steroid dose and regime specified
- Comparator = Patients receiving placebo

- Outcome = All Cause 60 day mortality
- Statistics = Absolute 20% reduction of mortality from an expected baseline of 40%, with a statistical power of 85%

The incomplete hypothesis is: Do steroid work in ARDS

The Complete hypothesis is: In persistent (7-28 days) ARDS (defined as ...), compared to placebo, do steroids (MPS regime of 2 mg/kg loading, 2 mg/kg/day for 14 days, 0.5mg/kg BD for 7 days), result in a (20% absolute) reduction in (all cause 60 day) mortality (compared to an expected 40% in placebo group) (with statistical power of 85%).

First read only the large font to get the basic question. Then read it with all specific details (in the small font in the brackets). After reading this carefully, it becomes clear that the incomplete hypothesis could lead to many different answers, but the complete hypothesis is specific and testable.

Step 2: Check that the methods are appropriate and sound

There is a checklist one needs to go through in the methods section to ensure that the study is actually capable of reaching an accurate and reliable conclusion. These are

1. Did the study ask a clearly focused question
2. Were participants appropriately randomized
3. Were all the participants accounted for at its conclusion
4. Were patients analyzed in the groups to which they were randomized
5. Were participants, staff, and study personnel blinded
6. Were the groups similar at the start of the study
7. Except for the experimental interventions, were participants in both groups treated in the same way?
8. Did the study have enough participants
9. How precise are the results
10. Were all important outcomes considered
11. Can the results be applied by you locally

Step 3: Go straight to the Tables and Figures

Usually the first 2-3 tables give patient data in both groups and the treatment received and observations made. The aim of these tables is to see that the patients were equivalent in both groups, and to see that the treatments were effective.

Figure 7, from the adrenaline vs. noradrenaline + dobutamine study, is an example of a flow chart that shows how many patients were screened, randomized, treated and followed up. One notes that more than 1500 patients were screened but only 330 were studied. The larger the proportion of patients enrolled, the more the study population represents the general ICU population with that disease. One also notes that all the patients enrolled were followed up to complete analysis. The lower the percentage followed up to completion, the less reliable the conclusion.

Table 2 below from the NICE study is an example that shows that after randomization, both patient groups had similar characteristics.

Looking at the tables and the figures sometimes gives one a more accurate idea than the text. For example in a BP target in trauma study, the targets were MBP of 50 vs. 65, but a look at the table shows that the MBP was nearly identical in both groups (Table 3).

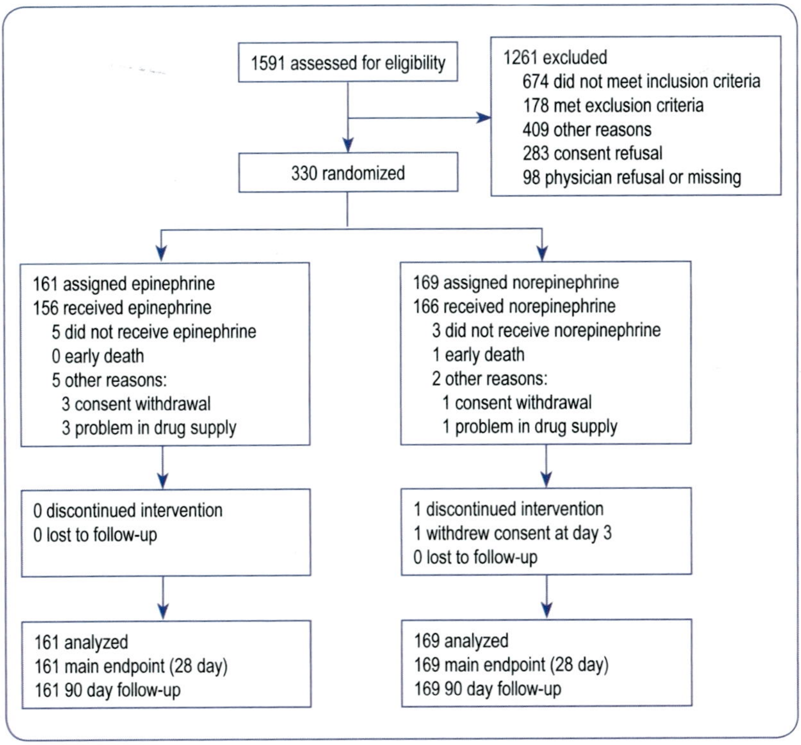

Figure 7. Flow chart that shows how many patients were screened, randomized, treated and followed up

Table 2. Patient Baseline Characteristics		
Variable	Intensive Glucose Control	Conventional Glucose Control
Age — yr	60.4±17.2	59.9±17.1
Female sex — no./total no. (%)	1128/3016 (37.4)	1079/3014 (35.8)
Weight — kg	80.7±21.4	80.9±21.2
Body-mass index†	27.9±7.7	28.0±7.2
Interval from ICU admission to randomization — hr	13.4±7.6	13.4±7.7
Reason for ICU admission — no./total no. (%)		
Operative	1112/3015 (36.9)	1121/3014 (37.2)
Nonoperative	1903/3015 (63.1)	1893/3014 (62.8)
Location before ICU admission — no./total no. (%)		
Emergency department	718/3015 (23.8)	749/3014 (24.9)
Hospital floor (or ward)		
Without previous ICU admission	640/3015 (21.2)	618/3014 (20.5)
With previous ICU admission	42/3015 (1.4)	30/3014 (1.0)
Another ICU	125/3015 (4.1)	102/3014 (3.4)
Another hospital	445/3015 (14.8)	453/3014 (15.0)
Operating room		
After emergency surgery	682/3015 (22.6)	671/3014 (22.3)
After elective surgery	363/3015 (12.0)	391/3014 (13.0)
APACHE II score	21.1±7.91	21.1±8.3
Blood glucose level — mg/dl	146±52.3	144±49.1
Organ failure or dysfunction — no./total no. (%)		
Respiratory		
Dysfunction (SOFA score, 1–2)	1207/2993 (40.3)	1222/2990 (40.9)
Failure (SOFA score, 3–4)	1526/2993 (51.0)	1521/2990 (50.9)
Coagulatory		
Dysfunction (SOFA score, 1–2)	947/2987 (31.7)	874/2989 (29.2)
Failure (SOFA score, 3–4)	128/2987 (4.3)	137/2989 (4.6)
Hepatic		
Dysfunction (SOFA score, 1–2)	831/2807 (29.6)	834/2802 (29.8)
Failure (SOFA score, 3–4)	70/2807 (2.5)	50/2802 (1.8)
Cardiovascular		
Dysfunction (SOFA score, 1–2)	583/3011 (19.4)	614/3012 (20.4)
Failure (SOFA score, 3–4)	1726/3011 (57.3)	1695/3012 (56.3)
Renal		
Dysfunction (SOFA score, 1–2)	1042/2981 (35.0)	1071/2974 (36.0)
Failure (SOFA score, 3–4)	249/2981 (8.4)	228/2974 (7.7)

Table 3. Intraoperative BP in trauma patients

	MAP = 50 mmHg				MAP = 65 mmHg				
	n	Mean	SD	CI	*n*	Mean	SD	CI	*P*
Temperature (°C)	29	35.1	1.5	34.6–35.7	36	34.7	1.5	34.2–35.3	0.32
SBP (mmHg)	42	96.7	18.4	91.0–102.4	46	100.6	19.5	94.8–106.3	0.34
DBP (mmHg)	41	50.6	8.7	47.8–53.3	45	54.3	1.6	51.2–57.4	0.08
MAP (mmHg)	42	64.7	11.7	61.0–68.3	46	68.5	12.9	64.7–72.3	0.15
MAP, first 30 min (mmHg)	42	64.6	11.7	61.0–68.3	46	67.7	12.6	64.3–71.5	0.23
Duration at MAP <65 (min)	42	42.9	35	32.0–53.8	46	31.5	29.5	22.8–40.3	0.10

DBP, diastolic blood pressure; CI, confidence interval.

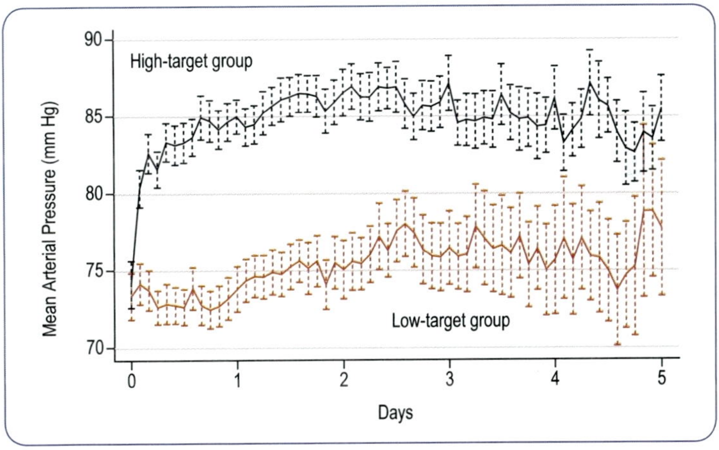

Figure 8. Blood Pressure during study

In the SEPSISPAM study, the target BP was 65 -70 vs. 80-85. A look at the actual BP (Figure 8) show that though they were different in both groups, they were higher than the targets.

The most important table or figure is the one that gives the primary outcome. This tells the reader the difference in outcomes in the two groups and whether this difference was a random observation, or could be attributed to the intervention or therapy. The primary end point could be shown as a figure or a table. Table 4 below shows similar mortality at different time points in the study that compared adrenaline to noradrenaline + dobutamine.

Table 4. All Cause mortality rates			
	Epinephine (n = 161)	Norepinephrine plus dobutamine (n = 169)	P
At day 7	40 (25%)	34 (20%)	0.30
At day 14	56 (35%)	44 (26%)	0.08
At day 28	64 (40%)	58 (34%)	0.31
At discharge from intensive care	75 (47%)	75 (44%)	0.69
At discharge from hospital	84 (52%)	82 (49%)	0.51
At day 90	84 (52%)	85 (50%)	0.73

Data are number of death (%).

Figure 9a and b below shows the mortality as a curve from the FEAST study and shows that the mortality was lower in the group that got no fluids at 48 hours and at 28 days.

The next tables and figure give similar information for the other endpoints.

Other tables show the effect on subgroups. The first example (Figure 10) shows that the adverse effects of saline or albumin bolus in the FEAST study persisted across all subgroups.

Figure 11 is from a trial comparing dopamine to noradrenaline in different forms of shock. It shows that though the overall outcomes were similar, noradrenaline appeared to be better in the subgroups of patients with cardiogenic shock.

We have shown a large number of these tables and figures in the chapter on the use of EBM for standard ICU therapies. Reading the paper or a chapter primarily through the figures and tables will give a better idea of the data than simply reading the text.

Step 4 and 5: Make your own interpretation and then read the text in detail

Having come to a tentative conclusion, it is worth then reading the full results and discussion section and seeing if there are any additional aspects or factors that affect the primary interpretation.

Step 6: Make a final interpretation of the study

At this point one should systematically go over the following issues. Is the primary end point positive? If yes, is it worth using the studied therapy on a routine basis. Are any of the secondary endpoints positive? If so, regardless of the primary end point, one should question

A Mortality at 48 Hours

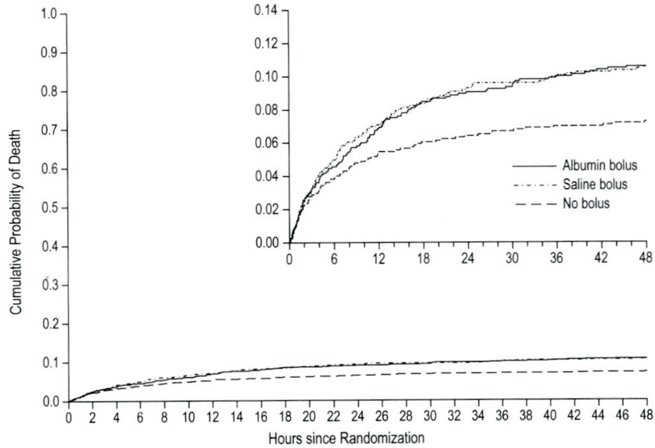

	Hr 1			Hr 2			Hr 3			Hr 4			Hr 5–8			Hr 9–24			Hr 24–48		
	Albumin bolus	Saline bolus	No bolus	Albumin bolus	Saline bolus	No bolus	Albumin bolus	Saline bolus	No bolus	Albumin bolus	Saline bolus	No bolus	Albumin bolus	Saline bolus	No bolus	Albumin bolus	Saline bolus	No bolus	Albumin bolus	Saline bolus	No bolus
No. at Risk	1050	1047	1044	1037	1033	1030	1024	1018	1021	1016	1010	1015	1010	1001	1011	992	980	996	954	945	975
Died	13	12	14	13	15	9	8	7	6	6	9	4	17	20	14	38	34	20	16	13	9
%	1.2	1.1	1.3	1.3	1.5	0.9	0.8	0.7	0.6	0.6	0.9	0.4	1.7	2.0	1.4	3.8	3.5	2.0	1.7	1.4	0.9

B Mortality at 4 Weeks

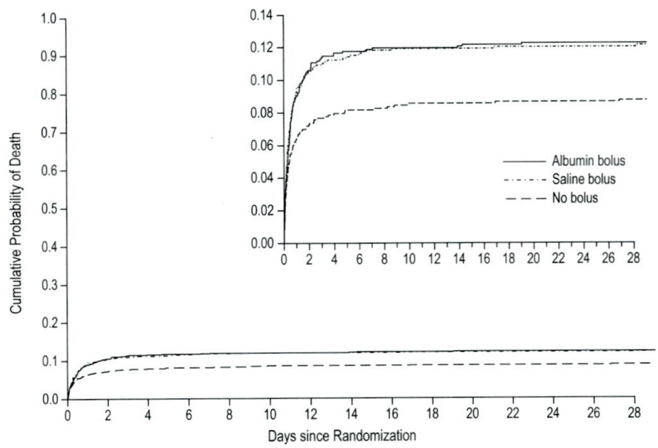

	Day 1			Day 2			Day 3–7			Day 8–14			Day 1 5–21			Day 21–28		
	Albumin bolus	Saline bolus	No bolus	Albumin bolus	Saline bolus	No bolus	Albumin bolus	Saline bolus	No bolus	Albumin bolus	Saline bolus	No bolus	Albumin bolus	Saline bolus	No bolus	Albumin bolus	Saline bolus	No bolus
No. at Risk	1050	1047	1044	954	945	975	914	917	947	901	909	940	899	902	933	897	901	934
Died	95	97	67	16	13	9	11	7	7	2	6	2	2	1	4	2	1	1
%	9.0	9.3	6.4	1.7	1.4	0.9	1.2	0.8	0.7	0.2	0.7	0.2	0.2	0.1	0.4	0.2	0.1	0.2

Figure 9a and 9b. Mortality Rates.

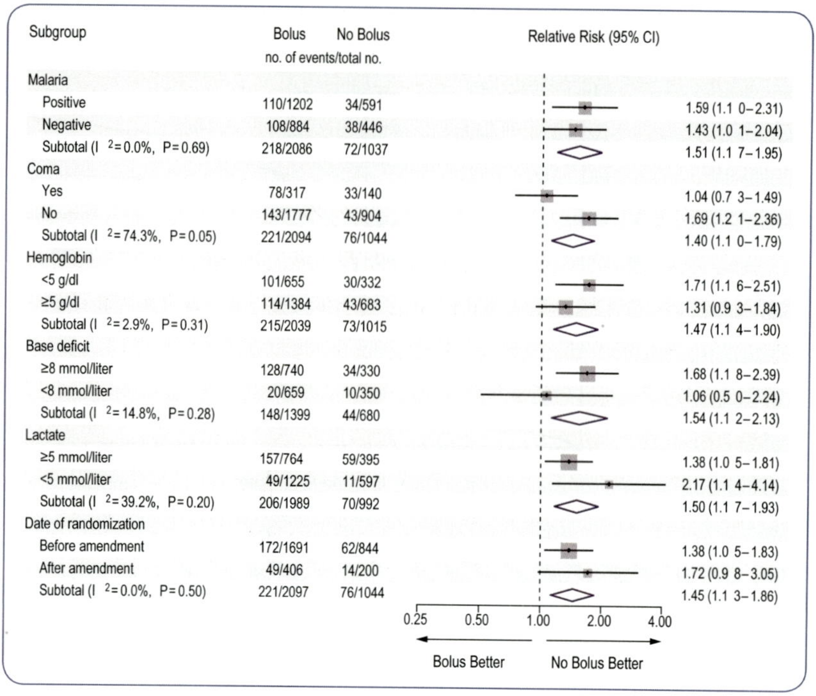

Figure 10. Mortality in Prespecified Sub groups.

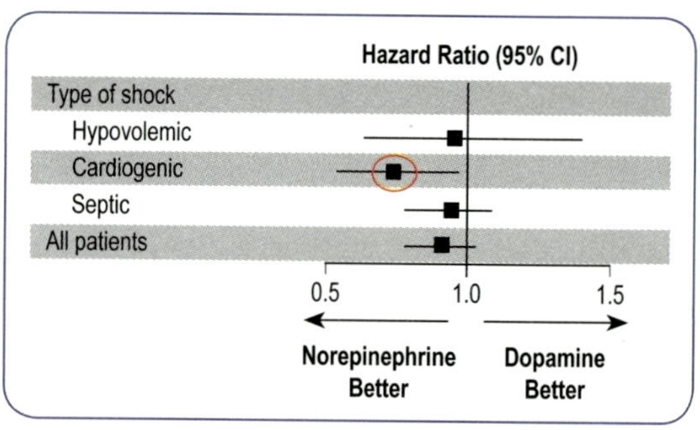

Figure 11. Predefined Sub group outcomes.

if the therapy is still worth using regularly. For example, in the FACTT study, mortality was unchanged, but duration of ventilation was less, so it is worth being restrictive with fluids in ARDS. Next look at the subgroup and post hoc analysis, and see if there are any advantages in the treatment group. One needs to be cautious in giving too much weight to these, but one should be aware of the potential advantages of the therapy in these analyses.

In a positive trial the next step is to see the magnitude of the effect by checking the relative and absolute risk reduction, and also calculating the numbers to treat. Once the above analysis is done, the reader should be in a position to make an informed decision about whether the therapy under study is worth using in his/her patients.

Summary

Large clinical trials with clinical endpoints are the most reliable method we currently have to evaluate if our therapies are effective. When reading an RCT, first identify the hypothesis clearly in terms of patients, interventions, comparators, outcomes and statistics. Then run through a quick checklist to confirm the methods are sound. Go over the tables to check the details of the population studied and the immediate effect intervention offered (e.g. blood pressure for vasoactive drugs and blood sugar for insulin). Then look at the tables and figures that evaluate the primary and secondary endpoints, and later the tables with the subgroup and post hoc analysis. Put it all together and decide if the therapy is effective and worth using in your patients.

Meta-Analysis: How to read

A Meta-analysis or systematic review is essentially a mathematical or statistical summary of multiple studies. PRISMA or Preferred Reporting Items for Systematic Reviews and Meta-Analyses (http://www.prisma-statement.org) comprehensively reviews the subject.

A cynic once compared the following scenario to a meta-analysis

Town Name: Statistics-ville

- Population: 10,000
- Average age: 35
- Height above sea level: 2,500 feet
- Average annual income: $ 15,000
- Average weight of population: 150 pounds.

Therefore, the average value of Statistics-ville is 5,537

There is an element of truth in this. Just combining data is not meta-analysis. The reliability of a meta-analysis can only be as good as the studies it includes, and of the methods it uses to draw conclusions. This is well shown (Figure 12) in a meta-analysis of the use of beta-blockers peri-operatively. (Reference cited in Chapter 9-Pitfall 6). If one takes one set

Study or subgroup	Beta-blocker Events	Total	Events	Total	Weight	Risk ratio M–H, Random, 95% CI
Secure trials		5264		5265	78.3%	1.27 [1.01, 1.60]
Non-secure trials		952		586	21.7%	0.42 [0.15, 1.23]

Test for subgroup differences; $Chi^2 = 3.91$, df = 1 ($P = 0.05$), $I^2 = 74.4\%$

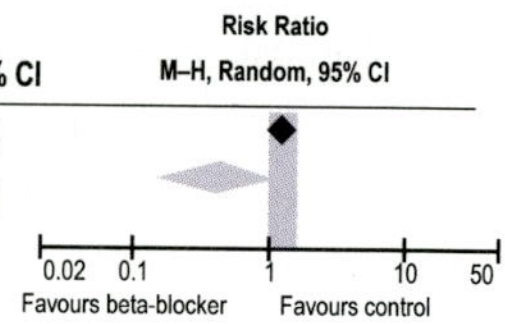

Figure 12. Difference in outcomes depending on studies chosen for the meta-analysis.

of "secure" studies, beta-blockers increased mortality, but if one takes another group of "non-secured" or fraudulent trials, beta-blockers appear protective.

The first step is to define the question or hypothesis one is planning to investigate. The next step is to search for studies that address this question. As discussed earlier, the more focused the hypothesis, the more uniform will be the selected studies. But, there will inevitably be variations between the studies. For example, if one is looking at steroids and mortality in ARDS, it is exceedingly unlikely that all studies will study the same dose, timing and duration of steroids. Similarly some may report ICU mortality, while others could report 7 day, 28 day, 60 day or hospital mortality. The investigator must select studies that are uniformly similar, though this will obviously limit the number of trials that will finally get included. The search method and inclusion criteria are usually discussed in the methods section. Bias in selecting articles will obviously affect the interpretation.

As in reading an RCT, once the hypothesis is focused, and the methods are sound, the story of that meta-analysis is best read by going straight to the Forest Plot, rather than by reading the text.

If there are multiple Forest Plots, first go to the one that looks at the primary outcome. In the case of COPD and NIV, this may be multiple outcomes such as mortality, reintubation, LOS on ventilator, LOS in ICU, and tolerance of therapy. Sometimes, the primary outcome may be a composite of selected individual outcomes. The steps while reading a Forest Plot are

1. See the list of studies.
2. Look at the rate of events in the treatment and control group.
3. Look at the Risk Ratio and 95% CI of each study
4. Look at the test for heterogeneity
5. See if a fixed or random effect model is selected
6. See the weightage calculation for each study (Total = 100%)
7. Look at the actual plot for each study
8. Look at the composite RR and 95% CI and decide of the intervention is effective or not.

The Forrest Plot below (Figure 13) is from Lightowler *et al.* NIV in COPD. Meta-analysis BMJ 2003. This particular one looks at the composite primary end-point of Mortality, Intubation and Intolerance to Treatment. We will use it to go through the above steps.

Step 1: See the list of studies.

The column on the immediate left lists seven studies starting with Avdeev and ending with Plant.

Step 2: Look at the rate of events in the treatment and control group.

The second column on the left gives this information. In this example, in the Avdeev study, 7/29 in the treatment arm and 12/29 in the control arm met the composite end point. This obviously means that the NIV arm had less events of mortality, intubation or intolerance of therapy.

Step 3: Look at the Risk Ratio and 95% CI of each study

The far right column gives this information. In this example, in the Avdeev study, the RR is 0.58 and the 95% CI is 0.27-1.27. A RR of 0.58 means that the risk of reaching the endpoint in the treatment arm was 58% of that of reaching the endpoint in the control arm. The 95%

Study	NPPV	Usual medical care	Weight (%)	Risk ratio (fixed 95% CI)
Avdeev et al 1998	7/29	12/29	11.2	0.58 (0.27 to 1.27)
Barbe et al 1996	4/14	0/10	0.5	6.60 (0.39 to 110.32)
Bott et al 1993	5/30	13/30	12.1	0.38 (0.16 to 0.94)
Brochard et al 1995	12/43	33/42	31.1	0.36 (0.21 to 0.59)
Celikel et al 1998	1/15	6/15	5.6	0.17 (0.02 to 1.22)
Dikensoy et al 2002	4/19	7/17	6.9	0.51 (0.18 to 1.45)
Plant et al 2000	22/118	35/118	32.6	0.63 (0.39 to 1.00)
Total (95% CI)	55/268	106/261	100	0.51 (0.38 to 0.67)

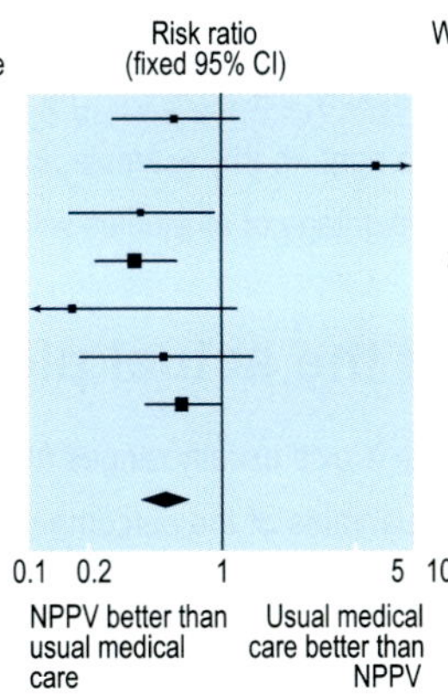

Test for heterogeneity: χ^2=7.59, df=6, P=0.27

Test for overall effect: Z=-4.82, P<0.0001

Figure 13. Forrest Plot for NIV in COPD studies.

CI of 0.27-1.27 means that if one were to perform similar study infinite times, in 95% of those studies the RR values would fall between 0.27 and 1.27.

Step 4: Look at the test for heterogeneity

This is given at the lower left corner of the figure. This reflects the similarity or differences of the population studied in the included studies. The more similar the results of the various trials, the more likely the cohort studied were similar, and the more varied the results between the trials, the more likely the populations studied were varied or different. In this case the value was 0.27. A value of 0 suggests a very homogenous cohort in all the studies, while a value of 1 suggests marked heterogeneity between the cohorts of patients in the various studies.

Step 5: See if a fixed or random effect model was used

The choice depends on the degree of heterogeneity. This information will be given above the actual plots. If there is low heterogeneity, the fixed effect model is used and if there is high heterogeneity, the variable effect model is used. In this example, because this was low (0.27) a fixed model was used.

Step 6: Look at the weightage for each study

In a fixed effects model this will depend on the number of patients and the number of events, with the outliers being given less weightage. In a random effects model, the weightage is dependent on the number of patients and the number of events and therefore more balanced. The weightage is used to modify the 95% CI. The weightage for each study is given in the second column from the right. In this example, in the Avdeev study the weightage was 11.2%. Note that the total weightage of all studies will be 100%.

Step 7: Look at the actual plot for each study

On the plot, the value on the X axis usually ranges from 0.1-10 with 1 placed in the middle. This value of 1 denotes equal rates of the outcome measure in both treatment and control groups. For each study, the point/line or the center of the box gives the risk reduction (RR), the size of the bars or "whiskers" give the weighted 95% CI and the size of the box denotes the relative weightage of that study. The RR gives an idea of the effect of the treatment and

95% CI tells us how reliable that number is. A RR point on either side of 1 favors either the treatment or the control group and this information is given below the X axis. In this Forest Plot, to the left of 1 (0.01-0.99) suggests that the NIV patients are doing better, and to the right of 1 (1.01-10), suggests that the controls are doing better. In this example, in terms of RR, it can be seen that in 6 of 7 trials the NIV group did better than the controls in terms of the composite outcome. However, in terms of the whiskers it can be seen that only in 2 of the 7 trials were the weighted 95% CI not touching or crossing the 1 mark. Current statistical thought is that if the 95% CI crosses 1, then the observation is more likely to be a random observation than a reliable treatment effect. This means that only in two of the 7 trials can we assume that the benefit was actually due to NIV and not simply a random observation.

Step 8: Look at the composite RR and 95% CI

This is denoted by the diamond shaped marker at the bottom of the plot. The further it is from the 1 line, the more effective the treatment, in this case, NIV. The lateral two tips of the diamond represent the weighted 95% CI and one need to see if this touches or crosses the 1 line. In this NIV meta-analysis it does not. The further from the 1 line the middle of the diamond, the greater the treatment effect. The further from the 1 line the lateral edge of the diamond, the more reliable the statistic. In this example we can conclude that there were 7 studies. In 6, the outcome (composite of mortality, intubation and intolerance to treatment) was less in the NIV group. In only two was the difference statistically significant. But putting all the data together, we can infer that NIV reliably decreased incidence of the composite endpoint compared to conventional treatment.

Before accepting the result of a meta-analysis, one needs to review the reliability of the study selection process. Two clues that the results of a meta analysis may not be reliable are the degree of heterogeneity, & the possibility of a publication bias. The former can be seen in the test of heterogeneity as explained above. A publication bias refers to the observation that negative studies tend to be published less frequently than positive ones. This may be because academic authors are less enthusiastic in submitting these studies. It could be that pharma would prefer not to submit data that suggest that their drug is ineffective. And journal editors tend to select studies that are positive as these are perceived as being more important. The possibility of publication bias can be judged by looking at the funnel plot (see figure 13). Each "dot" represents a study. Those at the top closer to the line are the larger studies, and hence more likely to be uniform, while those at the bottom are scattered as they represent smaller studies with mare variable results. The line from the top of the funnel plot to the X-axis represents the measured average effect. Those on one side of this line represent studies that favor the intervention & on the other side favor the control group (compared to the mean effect). If most of the dots are on one side of the line, it suggests that there is a potential publication bias in that there seem to be more published positive than negative studies. In this situation, one needs to be careful about accepting the results.

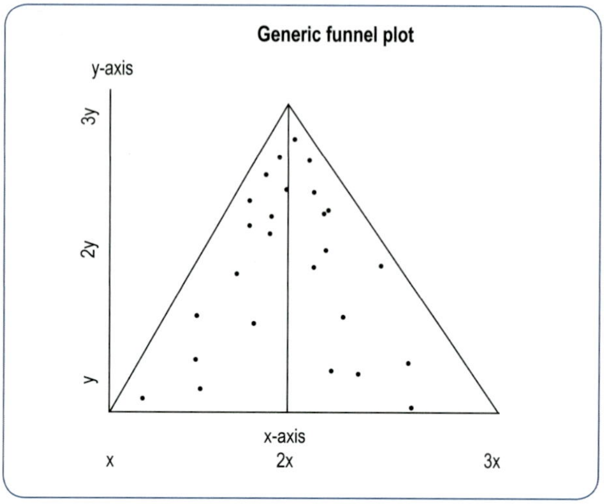

Figure 13. A Generic Funnel Plot Each dot is one study. The Y-axis represents the number of participants in the study. The higher the dot, the larger the study. The line on the X-axis shows the average effect of the drug. The distribution of the dots on either side of the line reflects the publication bias. In this example, the dots are equally distributed & this suggests absence of a publication bias.

In the final analysis, a meta-analysis can only be as reliable as the papers it evaluates, and there are many examples of meta-analysis of small studies giving opposite results from subsequent large RCTs. Still these meta-analyses allow one to get a sense of the summary of the available data.

The Limitations and Flaws of EBM

One of the most cited papers in the recent literature is the Ioannidis paper titled "Why Most Published Research Findings Are False".[1] This was one of many questioning the foundations of the methods used in contemporary EBM, in medicine in general,[2,3] in ICU[4] and even in satire.[5] This skepticism then appeared in the lay press.[6]

We list the limitations and flaws in EBM under the following categories:

- Absence of mathematical or statistical rigor
- Getting the initial assumptions wrong

- One P value does not fit all
- A relook at the concept of Randomness
- An Alternate Model: Bayesian Analysis

We finally explore the possibility that there is a fundamental error in EBM based on *P* values and frequency statistics, rendering most of our research unreliable.

Absence of mathematical or statistical rigor

In medicine and mathematics, there is a need for rigor. A single error in a single step can lead to an erroneous conclusion. Since most clinicians are not mathematicians or statisticians, they would invariably miss technical errors. For example, below is a mathematical "proof" that 1 =2.

1. Let a = b
2. Multiply both sides by a
   $\rightarrow a^2 = ab$
3. Add $a^2 - 2ab$ to both sides
   $\rightarrow a^2 + (a^2 - 2ab) = ab + (a^2 - 2ab)$
   $\rightarrow 2\ (a^2 - ab) = a^2 - ab$
4. Divide both sides by $a^2 - ab$
   $\rightarrow 2 = 1$

What is the error? In this case it is an erroneous use of the basic rules of mathematics. In this particular example we started with "a=b", and then introduced "a^2- ab". This "a^2- ab" = 0 and the rules for 0 are different. You cannot divide by 0. It is mathematically impermissible. In step 4 we introduce the mistake and reach the wrong conclusion. Most of us clinicians will need this error pointed out to us, as we do not have the academic background to spot it. In a similar way, an introduction of a single error can led to wrong conclusions, and occasionally a widely used wrong clinical practice. In the late 1980s and early 90s, the concept of "delivery dependent oxygen consumption" was used in resuscitating patients. This concept evolved from the observation than when we increased oxygen delivery (DO_2), we noted there was more oxygen consumption (VO_2). Both were measured and calculated using the data from the pulmonary artery catheter, the hemoglobin and the arterial and mixed venous saturation. At some point, statisticians pointed out that the whole relation between VO_2 and DO_2 might be explained purely by "mathematical coupling" and the observation may have nothing to do with physiology. The intensive care community took a long time to get to grips with this possible error, even though basic physiology textbooks such as Guyton teach that it's the VO_2 that dictates the DO_2, not the other way around.

Getting the Initial Assumptions Wrong

In every RCT, we start with two assumptions or guesses and use this for the power calculation. We estimate the baseline mortality and select a minimum meaningful effect. Based on this, we pick the minimum number of patients to study. If either of these guesses turns out wrong (in the data later generated in the study), then the conclusion becomes unreliable. As an example, in the adrenaline vs. noradrenaline + dobutamine study;

The **Methods** first state

"We expected an all-cause mortality rate at day 28 of 60% in the epinephrine group. We calculated that we would need a sample size of 340 patients to be able to detect an absolute reduction of 20% in the mortality rate at day 28 with 95% probability".

The **Results** then show

"At day 28, there were 64 (40%) deaths in the epinephrine group and 58 (34%) deaths in the norepinephrine plus dobutamine group".

The **Discussion** goes on to add

"In fact, to test the hypothesis that the absolute difference observed between groups in the day 28 all-cause mortality rate was real, 5000 patients would be needed to show statistical significance with a 95% probability."

This shows if the initial assumptions had been different, and the subsequent sample size different, then this could have been a positive trial rather than a negative one.

One P Value Does Not Fit All

When the p value was introduced and explored by Fisher, Pearson and others, it was simply a pragmatic cutoff to allow some interpretations to be made from the data. Over a period of time the value of < 0.05 became entrenched in the collective psyche of the medical community, and a statistical based cutoff was interpreted as a yes/no answer. One has to be pragmatic and choose some cut-off, but to select one value to fit all clinical circumstances is silly. Some populations are large and some are small. Some events are common and some are very rare. Some have minimal clinical significance, and other have devastating implications for the patients. We obviously should have different degrees of certainty for different clinical situations, but as an academic community, we have settled, mostly unquestioningly, with the two cut-offs of < 0.05 and <0.001.

Just like a $P< 0.05$ is a pragmatic cut-off, so is the use of 95% CI. The same results could become positive or negative, if the investigator chooses to use higher or lower Confidence Intervals.

A Relook at the Concept of Randomness

The whole concept of *P* value based statistics is itself based on the assumption that the data is random. As we saw earlier, it was first described as *"If a random event has several equally likely outcomes, the chance of any individual outcome occurring is equal to the proportion of that outcome to all possible outcomes"*. If the assumption that the data is random is flawed, all subsequent calculations are flawed. An example often given to demonstrate the non-random nature of things involves numbers. There are 10 digits, 0-9. Larger numbers are made from these digits. If we take a totally random sample of numbers, say, all the numbers in this chapter, or this book, or todays' newspaper, or one's tax returns, we could reasonably assume that the first digit of each number would be equally randomly distributed between the 9 digits. There would be some skewing towards the earlier numbers. (In a set of numbers from 0-9, all digits appear equally but in a set from 1-20, the digit 1 appears more often, and so on.) Yet, Newcomb in 1881 showed that the distribution was not random and numbers starting with the digit 1 were vastly overrepresented. Bedford rediscovered this more than half a century later. He consistently found that digits starting with 1 made 30% of all numbers *in any random sample*, such as this book, and those starting with 2 accounted for 18%. Half of all numbers appearing in any so called random set, will start with either the digit 1 or 2. He found it so wide spread that he felt it was a universal law that he labeled as The Law of Anomalous Numbers. It is usually referred to as Bedford's Law.

The point of this example is to highlight that our initial assumption of an underlying randomness itself may be false, following which all the probability based calculations will be wrong. Even if the data is truly random, there may be an unequal distribution purely by chance, just like as a series of coin tosses can occasionally have a disproportionately larger number of heads or tails. This form of randomization failure can partly overcome by techniques like block randomization to account for seasonal and location factors. An early RCT comparing HD vs. CRRT (Mehta RL, MsDonald B, Gabbai F *et al.* A randomized clinical trial of continuous versus intermittent dialysis for acute renal failure Kidney International

(2001);60:1154-63) is an example of "randomization failure" Despite being randomized, the two groups had significantly different severity scores, and hence risk of death. In this trial, there was a higher ICU and hospital mortality with CRRT. However, since randomization had resulted in the CRRT arm having a higher predicted mortality than the HD, we cannot conclude that CRRT was inherently more dangerous.

An Alternate Model: Bayesian Analysis

Thomas Bayes theorem was published in 1726, 20 years after his death.[7] This theorem is based on the following concepts. There is no basic presumption of randomness. Before a study, each event has a probability. After an experiment or trial, that probability changes, depending on the results of the study.

Prior Information (before a trial)

x = Initial probability of an event in a given condition (e.g. CVA in DM)

New event/information (from the trial)

y = Probability of event in presence of condition (CVA with DM)

z = Probability of event in absence of condition (CVA without DM)

Bayes Theorem: xy / xy +z(1-x)

There is no controversy regarding the theorem itself, but its application was questioned because it was presumed that the selection of a value for a pre-test probability was too subjective. Bayes Factor can also be represented as likelihood ratios, and evaluating data this way may remove some of the flaws of frequency statistics.

Is there a Fundamental Flaw in EBM based on P values and frequency statistics?

Mathematical proof is a form of absolute or 100% proof. Even here there is a proviso, that the initial conditions or axioms remain true and unchanged. In the example given of the proof of Pythogarus' theorem, the proof is subject to the surface being flat. If part of the surface became stretched, the proof would not hold. Similarly in the chess puzzle, the proof is subject to two squares of the same color from opposite corners being removed, and the dominos covering exactly two squares. If either of these changed, the proof would no longer be valid.

There is a very fundamental flaw in P value based statistics,[8] and this makes its reliability questionable, which then leads to papers with provocative titles such as "Why Most Published

Research Findings Are False", "Randomized Controlled Trials: Important but Overrated?", "The Hazards of Evidence-Based Medicine", "Multicenter, randomized, controlled trials evaluating mortality in intensive care: doomed to fail?", "The Truth Wears Off" and even "Cigarette smoking: an underused tool in high-performance endurance training."

Essentially the flaw is 2 fold. The first can be simplified into two sentences. We first use concept A to derive the value of B. We then use the value of B to reject concept A. To go back to the example of tossing a coin 10 times. We first presume randomness so the probability of each toss landing on heads is 1/2 (P = 0.5). If we get an "extreme" value, say all 10 heads, we calculate the p as 1/1024 (P =0.00098). Based on the extreme value we "reject" out initial presumption that there is an equal chance of Heads and Tails. But if we reject our initial presumption, then the calculation of the p value of 0.00098 is itself based on a wrong assumption. The calculation of the P value of 0.00098 is correct *only* if the original value of a single toss is 0.5. The second part of the flaw is that the same P value is interpreted as two different and mutually independent things. One is the rarity of the post hoc observation and the other is that the rarity represents a pre hoc cut-off for a false positive value.

This fundamental flaw in the interpretation of the P value, leads many statisticians to tear their hair out at the medical world's unquestioning acceptance of stating a null hypothesis, doing frequency statistics using random samples, and then concluding that a $P < 0.05$ is evidence of "proof".

What used to be called judgment is now called prejudice, and what used to be called prejudice is now called a null hypothesis . . . it is dangerous nonsense (dressed up as the 'scientific method') and will cause much trouble before it is widely appreciated as such.

– A.W.F. Edwards, Statistician and Geneticist and protégé of R.A. Fisher

We can overcome this P value fallacy by framing the questions differently. Rather than state a null hypothesis and then reject or accept it, we can choose two competing hypothesis (e.g. adrenaline decreases mortality and adrenaline does not decrease mortality) and then see which of the two the statistics support or favour.

Conclusion

The EBM appendix started by looking at the evolution of science and knowledge, especially the concept of proof and noted that scientific proof is not absolute. Based on the probability of the observation we infer if treatments are effective or not, and then do further calculations to judge how effective they are. We then suggest a pragmatic way of reading an RCT or a meta-analysis by focusing on the data in the figures and the tables to guide the interpretation. The concluding section explores some flaws and limitations of our contemporary techniques used in EBM. Clinicians will be able to make informed decisions only if they appreciate both the strengths and weakness of the research they rely on.

"All models are wrong, Some models are useful"

– George EP Box (statistician)

At present, the most useful models we have are large RCTs and meta-analysis evaluating clinically meaningful end points. It is possible that in future we will find these quaint and flawed, but for now, we have no better way of evaluating the therapies we use on our patients.

References

1. John P. A. Ioannidis Why Most Published Research Findings Are False. *PLoS Medicine* 2005;2(8):696-701. www.plosmedicine.org
2. JF Boylan, BP Kavanagh, J Armitage Randomized controlled trials: important but overrated? *J R Coll Physicians Edinb* 2011;41:126–31.
3. Livingston EH, McNutt RA.. The Hazards of Evidence-Based Medicine. Assessing Variations in Care. *JAMA* 2011;306:762–63.
4. Ospina-Tascón GA1, Büchele GL, Vincent JL. Multicenter, randomized, controlled trials evaluating mortality in intensive care: doomed to fail? *Crit Care Med.* 2008 ;36(4):1311–22.
5. Kenneth A. Myers BSc Cigarette smoking: an underused tool in high-performance endurance training. *CMAJ* 2010;182(18):E867–869.
6. The New Yorker. Annals of Science. The Truth Wears Off. Is there something wrong with the scientific method? by Jonah Lehrer December 13, 2010.
7. Goodman SN. Toward Evidence-Based Medical Statistics. 2: The Bayes Factor Ann Intern Med 1999;130:1005–13.
8. Goodman SN. Toward Evidence-Based Medical Statistics. 1: The P Value Fallacy Ann Intern Med 1999;130:995–1004.

INDEX

A

B

C

D

E

F

G

H

I

L

M

N

O

P

R

S

T

V

W

TABLE OF CONTENTS